PSYCHOPHARMACOLOGY OF ANTIDEPRESSANTS

STEPHEN M. STAHL, MD, PhD

Director
Clinical Neuroscience Research Center
and
Adjunct Professor of Psychiatry
University of California
San Diego

Illustrations by
Nancy Muntner

Presented with the compliments of

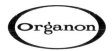

MARTIN DUNITZ

© Stephen M Stahl 1999

First published in the United Kingdom in 1997 by Martin Dunitz Ltd, 7–9 Pratt Street, London NW1 0AE

Reprinted with revises 1999

ISBN 1-85317-540-4

Composition by Scribe Design, Gillingham, Kent, UK
Printed and bound in Spain by Cayfosa

CONTENTS

Section 1: Neuroscientific Basis of Antidepressant Action

1. **Introduction**

2. **Monoamine Hypothesis of Depression**
   - monoamines
   - neurotransmitter receptors

3. **Three Key Neurotransmitter Systems**
   - mediators of antidepressant psychopharmacology
   - norepinephrine (noradrenaline)
   - dopamine
   - serotonin (5-hydroxytryptamine; 5HT)
   - norepinephrine–serotonin interactions

Section 2: Pharmacologic Mechanism of Action of Specific Antidepressant Drugs

4. **Classical Antidepressants: MAO Inhibitors and Tricyclic Antidepressants**

5. **The Serotonin Selective Reuptake Inhibitors**
   - fluoxetine
   - fluvoxamine
   - paroxetine
   - sertraline
   - citalopram

6. Other Neurotransmitter Mechanisms
– venlafaxine
– trazodone
– nefazodone
– bupropion
– mianserin
– mirtazapine

7. Antidepressant Summary
– matching pharmacologic profiles to patient profiles
– are two mechanisms better than one?

Section 3: For the Expert

8. Antidepressant Combinations and Augmentation Strategies for Difficult Cases

9. Cytochrome P450 and Antidepressant Drug Interactions

ACKNOWLEDGMENT

Figures in *Psychopharmacology of Antidepressants* are reproduced with permission from Stahl, S.M., *Essential Psychopharmacology* (Cambridge University Press, 1996), and from additional figures copyright Stephen M. Stahl, 1996.

CHAPTER 1

INTRODUCTION

This pocketbook is a series of visual lessons on the antidepressants. There are more than two dozen agents working by over six pharmacological mechanisms on three key neurotransmitter systems. The antidepressants discussed here are among the most widely prescribed agents in the world. Although these drugs are key members of a psychiatrist's therapeutic armamentarium, well over half of the prescriptions for antidepressants are written by non-psychiatric physicians. Thus, this class of drugs is of broad interest throughout all medical specialties.

This pocketbook is divided into three parts: the first part includes three chapters presenting important basic science concepts helpful in understanding not only the biological basis of depression, but also the three key neurotransmitter systems which are thought to mediate the therapeutic actions of virtually every known antidepressant agent. These systems are norepinephrine (noradrenaline), dopamine and serotonin (5-hydroxy-tryptamine; 5HT).

The second section deals with all known classes of antidepressant drugs, and utilizes pharmacological concepts to explain not only how individual agents mediate their antidepressant actions, but also how they mediate their side effects. The agents covered include the classical tricyclic antidepressants (TCAs) and MAO (monoamine oxidase) inhibitors, as well as the newer agents. One of the most important groups of antidepressants is the serotonin selective reuptake inhibitors (SSRIs). The SSRIs have revolutionized the use of safe drug therapies not only for depression, but also for a wide range of psychiatric disorders from anxiety disorders, such as obsessive compulsive disorder, and panic disorder to eating disorders such as bulimia. Other newer antidepressant agents include drugs acting on multiple neurotransmitter systems and receptors simultaneously, such as venlafaxine, nefazodone and mirtazapine. As some drugs are not approved in all countries, the more widely marketed agents will be emphasized.

Given the plethora of options, selection of a specific antidepressant for an individual patient can be a daunting (or largely random) decision. A series of visual lessons in the second section profiles the various individual antidepressant agents by their distinct pharmacological mechanisms of action. The value of this information is that it can assist a prescriber in making a drug selection from rational predictions of tolerability and efficacy for individual patients. The approach is to match pharmacological profiles of the drugs to symptom profiles of patients. Side effects and therapeutic effects from unsatisfactory trials with previously administered antidepressant drugs should also be taken into consideration.

The final section is for the expert who wishes to pursue or avoid drug combinations to improve tolerability, boost efficacy, or avoid toxic drug interactions.

The figures and diagrams are based largely upon the textbook *Essential Psychopharmacology* (Cambridge University Press, 1996), which the reader is encouraged to consult for further details and references.

CHAPTER 2

MONOAMINE HYPOTHESIS OF DEPRESSION

For over 30 years, the leading theory to explain the biological basis of depression has been the "monoamine hypothesis of depression." This theory proposes that depression is due to a deficiency in one or another of three biogenic monoamines, namely serotonin, norepinephrine (noradrenaline) and/or dopamine.

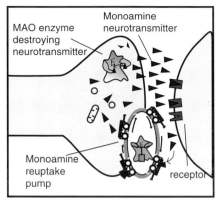

NORMAL STATE - NO DEPRESSION

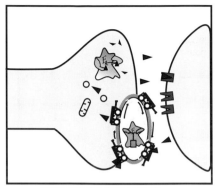

**DEPRESSION: CAUSED BY
NEUROTRANSMITTER DEFICIENCY**

FIGURE 2.1. This represents the normal state of a monoaminergic neuron, which is releasing its monoamine neurotransmitter at a normal rate, so there is no depression here. All the regulatory elements of the neuron are also normal: namely, the enzyme monoamine oxidase (MAO) which destroys the neurotransmitter; the monoamine reuptake pump which terminates the action of the neurotransmitter by sweeping it out of the synapse; and the postsynaptic receptors which react to the release of neurotransmitter.

FIGURE 2.2.   In the case of depression, the monoamine neurotransmitter is depleted, causing neurotransmitter deficiency.

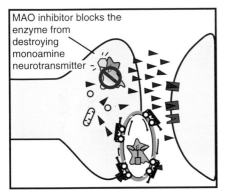

MAO inhibitor blocks the enzyme from destroying monoamine neurotransmitter

**INCREASE IN NEUROTRANSMITTERS
CAUSES RETURN TO NORMAL STATE**

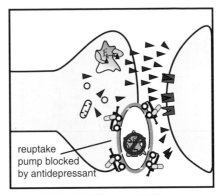

reuptake pump blocked by antidepressant

**INCREASE IN NEUROTRANSMITTERS
CAUSES RETURN TO NORMAL STATE**

FIGURE 2.3. MAO inhibitors act as antidepressants, since they block the enzyme MAO from destroying monoamine neurotransmitters, thus allowing them to accumulate. This accumulation theoretically reverses the prior neurotransmitter deficiency (see Figure 2.2) and relieves depression by returning the monoamine neuron to the normal state.

FIGURE 2.4. Tricyclic antidepressants act as antidepressants, since they block the neurotransmitter reuptake pump, thus causing neurotransmitter to accumulate. This accumulation theoretically reverses the prior neurotransmitter deficiency (see Figure 2.2) and relieves depression by returning the monoamine neuron to the normal state.

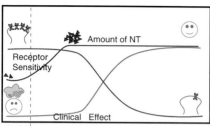

Antidepressant introduced

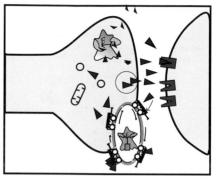

Normal functioning

FIGURE 2.5. This figure depicts the different time courses for three effects of antidepressant drugs, namely changes in mood, changes in neurotransmitters (NT) and changes in receptor sensitivity. Specifically, the amount of NT changes relatively rapidly after the antidepressant is introduced. However, the clinical effect is delayed, as is the down regulation of neurotransmitter receptor sensitivity. This temporal correlation of clinical effects with changes in receptor sensitivity has given rise to the hypothesis that changes in neurotransmitter receptor sensitivity may actually mediate the clinical effects of antidepressant drugs.

FIGURE 2.6. Monoamine receptor hypothesis of depression. This theory posits that an abnormality in the receptors for monoamine neurotransmitters leads to depression. Such a disturbance in neurotransmitter receptors may be itself caused by depletion of monoamine neurotransmitters. Depicted here is the normal monoamine neuron with the normal amount of monoamine neurotransmitter and the normal amount of correctly functioning monoamine receptors.

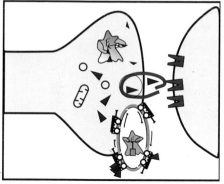

Decrease in NT

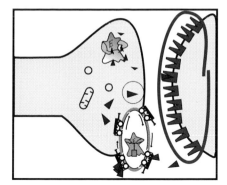

**Receptors up-regulate
due to lack of NT**

FIGURE 2.7. In this figure, monoamine neurotransmitter is depleted (see red circle), just as previously shown in Figure 2.2.

FIGURE 2.8. The consequences of monoamine neurotransmitter depletion of the previous Figure 2.7 is that the postsynaptic receptors abnormally up-regulate (indicated in red circle). This upregulation correlates with the production of the depressive illness, and is hypothetically linked to the cause of depression.

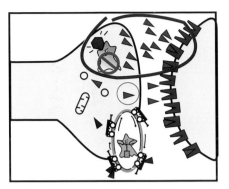

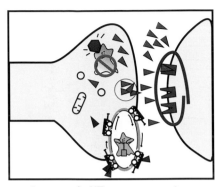

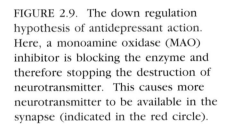

**MAO inhibitor tells the enzyme
to stop destroying NE**

**Increase in NT causes receptors
to down-regulate**

FIGURE 2.9. The down regulation hypothesis of antidepressant action. Here, a monoamine oxidase (MAO) inhibitor is blocking the enzyme and therefore stopping the destruction of neurotransmitter. This causes more neurotransmitter to be available in the synapse (indicated in the red circle).

FIGURE 2.10. The consequence of long-lasting blockade of MAO (monoamine oxidase) by an MAO inhibitor is for the neurotransmitter receptors to down regulate (indicated in the red circle). This correlates with the onset of anti-depressant action.

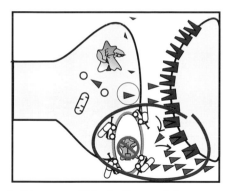

Antidepressant blocks the reuptake pump, causing more NT to be in the synapse

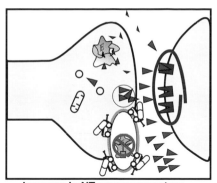

Increase in NT causes receptors to down-regulate

FIGURE 2.11. Here, a tricyclic antidepressant blocks the reuptake pump, causing more neurotransmitter to be available in the synapse (indicated in the red circle). This is very similar to what happens after MAO is inhibited (see Figure 2.9).

FIGURE 2.12. The consequence of long-lasting blockade of the reuptake pump by a tricyclic antidepressant is for the neurotransmitter receptors to down regulate (indicated in the red circle). This is the same outcome as with long-lasting blockade of MAO (see Figure 2.10), and also correlates with the onset of antidepressant action.

CHAPTER 3

THREE KEY NEUROTRANSMITTER SYSTEMS

This chapter presents the neurobiological basis of antidepressant action by explaining important aspects of three neurotransmitter systems in the central nervous system. The three neurotransmitter systems are:

- norepinephrine (also noradrenaline or NE)
- dopamine
- serotonin (also 5-hydroxytryptamine or 5HT).

A series of figures show how each neurotransmitter is synthesized and metabolized as well as how each interacts at various receptors. Finally, several diagrams explain the manner in which norepinephrine controls the release of serotonin, both by stimulating and by inhibiting serotonin release.

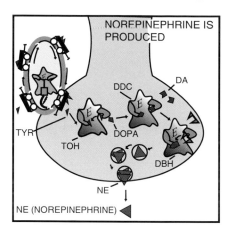

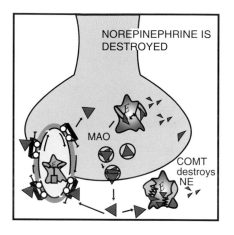

FIGURE 3.1. This figure shows how the neurotransmitter norepinephrine (or noradrenaline) (NE) is produced in noradrenergic neurons. This process starts with the amino acid precursor of NE, tyrosine (TYR), being transported into the nervous system from the blood by means of an active transport pump. This active transport pump for tyrosine is separate and distinct from the active transport pump for NE itself (see Figure 3.2). Once pumped inside the neuron, the tyrosine is acted upon by three enzymes in sequence: first, tyrosine hydroxylase (TOH), the rate limiting and most important enzyme in the regulation of NE synthesis. Tyrosine hydroxylase converts the amino acid tyrosine into di-hydroxy-phenyl-alanine (DOPA). The second enzyme then acts, namely, DOPA decarboxylase (DDC), which converts DOPA into dopamine (DA). The third and final NE synthetic enzyme, dopamine beta hydroxylase (DBH), converts DA into NE. NE is then stored in synaptic packages called vesicles until released by a nerve impulse.

FIGURE 3.2. Norepinephrine (nor-adrenaline) (NE) can also be destroyed by enzymes in the NE neuron. The principal destructive enzymes are monoamine oxidase (MAO) and catechol-O-methyl transferase (COMT). The action of NE can be terminated not only by enzymes which destroy NE, but also by a transport pump for NE which removes it from acting in the synapse without destroying it. This transport pump is separate and distinct from the transport pump for tyrosine used in carrying tyrosine into the NE neuron for NE synthesis (see Figure 3.1). The transport pump which terminates the synaptic action of NE is sometimes called the 'NE transporter' and sometimes the 'NE reuptake pump.' It is selective for NE and not for any other neurotransmitter (see also the dopamine transporter in Figure 3.6 and the serotonin transporter in Figure 3.9). The NE transporter is part of the presynaptic machinery where it acts like a vacuum cleaner whisking NE out of the synapse, off the synaptic receptors, and stopping its synaptic actions. Once inside the presynaptic nerve terminal, NE can either be stored again for subsequent reuse when another nerve impulse arrives, or it can be destroyed by NE destroying enzymes.

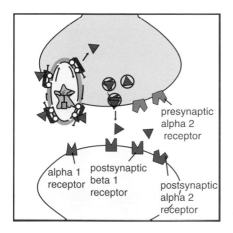

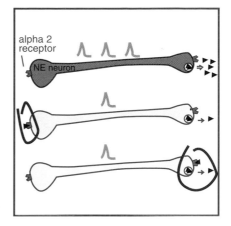

FIGURE 3.3. The noradrenergic neuron is regulated by a multiplicity of receptors for NE. Pictured here are the NE transporter, and several NE receptors, including alpha 1, alpha 2 and beta 1 adrenergic receptors. Three of these receptors are located on the postsynaptic neuron, including the beta 1 receptor and both the alpha 1 and the alpha 2 adrenergic receptors. Postsynaptic NE receptors generally act by recognizing when NE is released from the presynaptic neuron, and reacting by setting up a molecular cascade in the postsynaptic neuron, thereby causing neurotransmission to pass from the presynaptic neuron to the postsynaptic neuron.

The presynaptic alpha 2 receptor located on the NE terminal is important because it is an autoreceptor. That is, when the presynaptic alpha 2 receptor recognizes synaptic NE, it turns off further release of NE. Thus the presynaptic alpha 2 terminal autoreceptor acts as a brake for the NE neuron. Stimulating this receptor (i.e. stepping on the brake) stops the neuron from firing. This probably occurs physiologically to prevent over-firing of the NE neuron, since it can shut itself off once the firing rate gets too high and the autoreceptor becomes stimulated.

FIGURE 3.4. This figure shows that alpha 2 receptors exist both on the cell body (middle neuron) as well as on the axon terminal (bottom neuron) of the noradrenergic neuron. Thus, the NE neuron has two ways to turn itself off since alpha 2 receptors in both places act to slow neuronal impulse flow and inhibit the release of NE. Since NE turns off its own release with this receptor it is called an *auto*receptor.

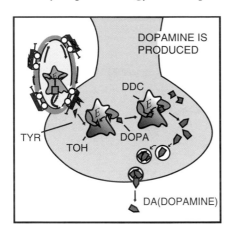

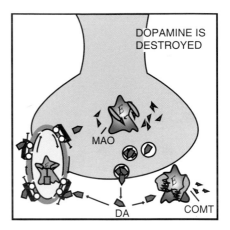

FIGURE 3.5.   Dopamine (DA) is produced in dopaminergic neurons from the precursor tyrosine (TYR), which is tranported into the neuron by an active transport pump, and then converted into DA by 2 out of 3 of the same enzymes which also synthesize norepinephrine (Figure 3.1). The DA synthesizing enzymes are tyrosine hydroxylase (TOH), which produces DOPA, followed by dopa decarboxylase (DDC), which produces DA.

FIGURE 3.6.   Dopamine (DA) is destroyed by the same enzymes which destroy norepinephrine (see Figure 3.2), namely monoamine oxidase (MAO) and catechol-O-methyl-transferase (COMT). The DA neuron has a presynaptic transporter (reuptake pump) which is unique for DA, but works analogously to the NE transporter (Figure 3.2).

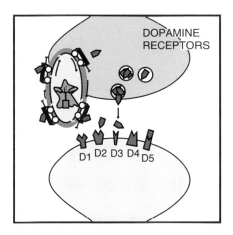

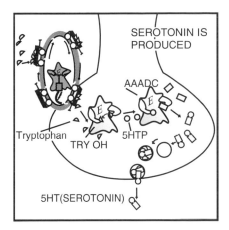

FIGURE 3.7.   Receptors for dopamine (DA) regulate dopaminergic neurotransmission. A plethora of dopamine receptors exist, including at least five pharmacological subtypes and several more molecular isoforms. Perhaps the most extensively investigated dopamine receptor is the dopamine 2 (D2) receptor, as it is stimulated by dopaminergic agonists for the treatment of Parkinson's Disease, and blocked by dopamine antagonist neuroleptics for the treatment of schizophrenia.

FIGURE 3.8.   Serotonin (5HT; 5-hydroxytryptamine) is produced from enzymes after the amino acid precursor tryptophan is transported into the serotonin neuron. The tryptophan transport pump is distinct from the scrotonin transporter (see Figure 3.9). Once transported into the serotonin neuron, tryptophan is converted into 5-hydroxytryptophan (5HTP) by the enzyme tryptophan hydroxylase (TRY OH). 5HTP is then converted into 5HT by the enzyme aromatic amino acid decarboxylase (AAADC). Serotonin is then stored in synaptic vesicles where it stays until released by a neuronal impulse.

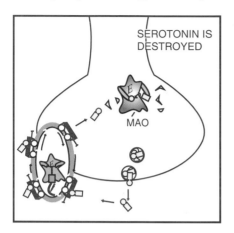

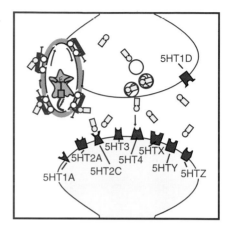

FIGURE 3.9.   Serotonin is destroyed by the enzyme monoamine oxidase (MAO), and converted into an inactive metabolite. The 5HT neuron has a presynaptic transport pump selective for serotonin called the serotonin transporter, analogous to the norepinephrine (NE) transporter in NE neurons (Figure 3.2) and to the DA transporter in DA neurons (Figure 3.6).

FIGURE 3.10.   Receptor subtyping for the serotonergic neuron has proceeded at a very rapid pace, with at least four major categories of 5HT receptors, each further subtyped depending upon pharmacologic properties or molecular properties. In addition to the serotonin transporter, there is a key presynaptic serotonin receptor (the 5HT1D receptor) and several postsynaptic serotonin receptors (5HT1A, 5HT1D, 5HT2A, 5HT2C, 5HT3, 5HT4 and many others denoted by 5HT X,Y and Z).

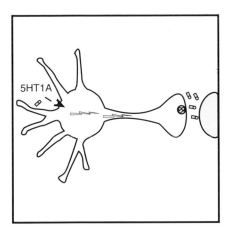

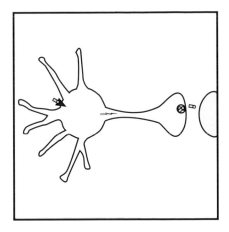

FIGURE 3.11.   Presynaptic 5HT1A receptors are autoreceptors, are located on the cell body and dendrites, and are therefore called somatodendritic autoreceptors.

FIGURE 3.12.   The 5HT1A somatodendritic autoreceptors depicted in Figure 3.11 act by detecting the presence of 5HT, and causing a shut down of 5HT neuronal impulse flow, depicted here as decreased electrical activity.

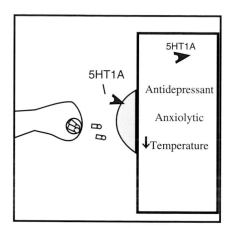

Table 3.1
Clinical tips about 5HT 1A receptors
CLINICALLY SIGNIFICANT CONSEQUENCES OF STIMULATING 5HT1A RECEPTORS
• antidepressant actions • anti-obsessive compulsive disorder properties • anti-panic and anti-social phobia properties • anti-bulimia properties

FIGURE 3.13.   Pharmacology of the 5HT1A receptor. This receptor has two forms: one presynaptic and one postsynaptic. The presynaptic receptor controls serotonin release, so when it is down regulated, it causes increased release of serotonin (also called disinhibition of the serotonin neuron), and thus, therapeutic effects in depression, anxiety disorders and eating disorders. The postsynaptic receptor may help send chemical signals from the serotonin neuron to other neurons, and also has a role in temperature regulation.

Thus, the presynaptic 5HT1A receptor contributes in a major way to the overall therapeutic profile of the SSRIs.

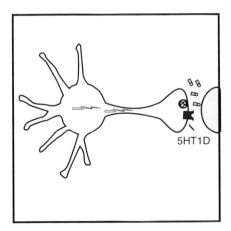

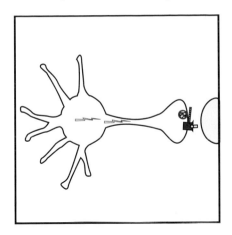

FIGURE 3.14.   Presynaptic 5HT1D receptors are also a type of autoreceptor, but are located on the presynaptic axon terminal, and are therefore called terminal autoreceptors.

FIGURE 3.15.   Presynaptic 5HT1D terminal autoreceptors act as regulators of 5HT release. If the 5HT1D receptor is stimulated, it blocks the release of 5HT.

Table 3.2
Clinical tips about 5HT1D receptors
CLINICALLY SIGNIFICANT CONSEQUENCES OF STIMULATING 5HT1D RECEPTORS
• anti-migraine actions

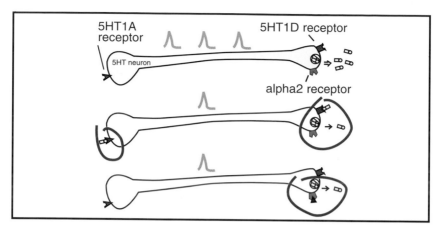

FIGURE 3.16.   All three receptors which can inhibit the release of serotonin are shown here. In the top neuron, the serotonin neuron is firing and serotonin is being released.

Shown are three presynaptic inhibitory autoreceptors: the first is the 5HT1A receptor on the left, which is located on the cell body and dendrites and is called a somatodendritic autoreceptor. This has already been shown in Figures 3.11 and 3.12. This receptor can inhibit both serotonin firing and serotonin release when serotonin occupies this receptor, as shown on the left hand portion of the middle neuron.

The second inhibitory receptor is the 5HT1D receptor located on the axon terminal on the right hand part of the upper neuron. This has already been shown in Figures 3.14 and 3.15. This receptor can inhibit serotonin release when serotonin occupies this receptor, as shown on the right hand portion of the middle neuron.

The third inhibitory receptor on the serotonin neuron is the presynaptic alpha 2 receptor on the axon terminal on the right hand part of these serotonin neurons. This receptor will be explained further in Figures 3.23–3.28. Here, it is shown that this alpha 2 receptor can inhibit serotonin release when norepinephrine (noradrenaline) occupies it (on the right hand portion of the bottom neuron.)

Thus, there are three ways to inhibit a serotonin neuron: by stimulating 5HT1A autoreceptors, 5HT1D autoreceptors or alpha 2 receptors. Since a *different* neurotransmitter, namely norepinephrine, is regulating serotonin, its alpha 2 heteroreceptor is called a *hetero*receptor rather than an autoreceptor (see also Figure 3.4).

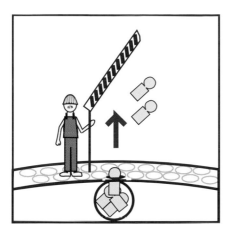

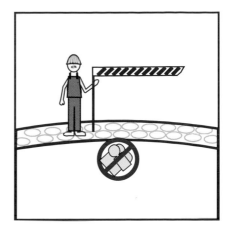

FIGURE 3.17.   When the three inhibitory receptors shown in Figure 3.16 are not occupied, the gates are open, and serotonin can be released.

FIGURE 3.18.   However, when any inhibitory autoreceptor or hetero-receptor is occupied by its neurotransmitter, it shuts off serotonin release by closing the gate. In this way, neurotransmitters can control the amount of their own release and prevent excessive amounts of release from occurring.

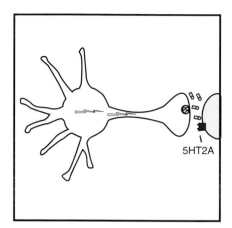

FIGURE 3.19.   A key postsynaptic regulatory receptor is the 5HT2A receptor.

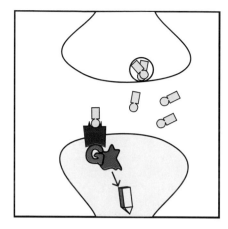

FIGURE 3.20.   When the postsynaptic 5HT2A receptor of Figure 3.19 is occupied by 5HT, it causes neuronal impulses in the postsynaptic neuron to be altered via the production of second messengers. Second messengers cause the production of intracellular chemicals called transcription factors. These transcription factors cause or block the expression of neuronal genes.

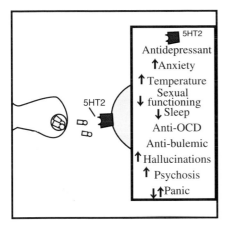

Table 3.3
Clinical tips about 5HT2 receptors

CLINICALLY SIGNIFICANT CONSEQUENCES OF STIMULATING 5HT2 RECEPTORS

- Agitation
- Akathisia
- Anxiety
- Panic attacks
- Insomnia
- Sexual dysfunction

FIGURE 3.21.   Although stimulation of the 5HT2 receptor by serotonin when antidepressants enhance serotonin release (i.e. when they disinhibit serotonergic neurons) may ultimately play a role in some of the therapeutic effects of serotonin selective reuptake inhibitors (SSRIs), they certainly seem to mediate several of the side effects of the SSRIs, in different pathways within the central nervous system. These are discussed in greater detail in chapter 5. The 5HT2 receptor and its A and C subtypes may mediate the effects of hallucinogens such as LSD. This receptor may also mediate changes in psychosis since blocking this receptor with the new designer antipsychotics such as risperidone and olanzapine improve psychosis.

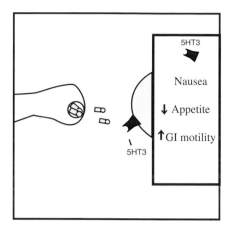

Table 3.4
Clinical tips about 5HT3 receptors

CLINICALLY SIGNIFICANT CONSEQUENCES OF STIMULATING 5HT3 RECEPTORS

- Nausea
- Gastrointestinal (GI) distress
- Diarrhoea
- Headache

FIGURE 3.22.   Stimulation of the 5HT3 receptor appears to be responsible for various gastrointestinal side effects of the SSRIs. These effects are mediated not only in central nervous system pathways such as the brainstem vomiting center and the pathway to hypothalamus, but also outside the brain in the gut itself, which also has 5HT3 receptors.

Table 3.5

Types of NE-5HT Interactions:

Presynaptic
    axo-axonic
    terminal alpha-2 autoreceptor

Postsynaptic
    axo-dendritic
    5-somatodendritic
    excitatory alpha-1 receptors

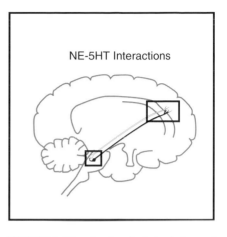

NE-5HT Interactions

Listed here are two important types of interactions between norepinephrine (noradrenaline) (NE) and serotonin (5-hydroxytryptamine) (5HT). The *presynaptic* interaction provides for NE to act like a *brake* to inhibit 5HT release. The *post-synaptic* interaction provides for NE to act like an *accelerator* to stimulate 5HT release.

FIGURE 3.23.   Anatomical depiction of NE-5HT interactions. These are described in Table 3.5 and are enlarged in Figures 3.24–3.28. The box at the left denotes the postsynaptic interaction between NE and 5HT (enlarged in Figures 3.24 and 3.25). This is an excitatory interaction.

The box at the right denotes the presynaptic interaction between NE and 5HT (enlarged in Figures 3.26 and 3.27). This is an inhibitory interaction.

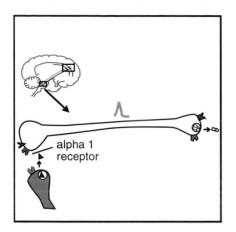

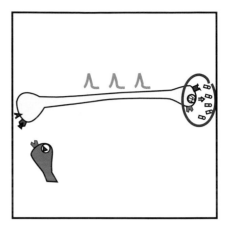

alpha 1
receptor

FIGURE 3.24.   Excitatory interaction between NE and 5HT: NE acting as an accelerator. When the 5HT neuron receives NE input postsynaptically at its cell body and dendrites, it is excitatory. That is, an NE signal from an NE neuron is received by an excitatory postsynaptic alpha 1 receptor on a 5HT neuron.

FIGURE 3.25.   When NE comes to the 5HT neuron on the left, it causes 5HT to be released from the axon terminal on the right. By this mechanism, NE enhances 5HT release.

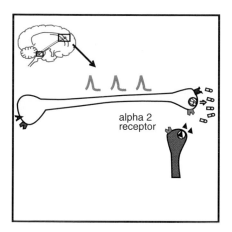

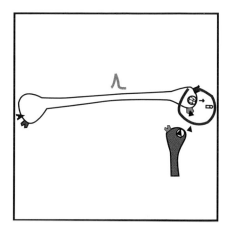

FIGURE 3.26.   Inhibitory interaction between NE and 5HT: NE acting as a brake. When the 5HT neuron receives NE input presynaptically at its axon terminal, it is inhibitory. That is, an NE signal from an NE neuron is received by an inhibitory presynaptic alpha 2 receptor on a 5HT neuron. This alpha 2 receptor is also called an alpha 2 heteroreceptor.

FIGURE 3.27.   When NE comes to the 5HT neuron on the right, it causes 5HT release to be inhibited from the axon terminal on the right. By this mechanism, NE blocks 5HT release.

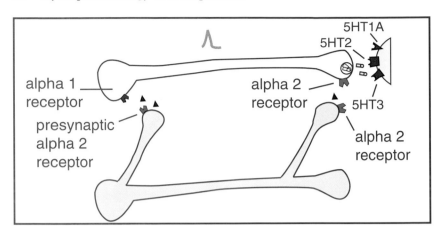

FIGURE 3.28. Integrated model of NE-5HT interactions. The accelerator shown on the left (mediated by alpha 1 receptors) and the brake on the right (mediated by alpha 2 heteroreceptors). This integrates the functions previously shown in Figures 3.23–3.27.

CHAPTER 4

CLASSICAL ANTIDEPRESSANTS: MAO INHIBITORS AND TRICYCLIC ANTIDEPRESSANTS

The first antidepressants were discovered 40 years ago by serendipity. Only much later was it determined that these early agents worked either by inhibiting the enzyme monoamine oxidase (MAO) or by blocking the reuptake of norepinephrine and serotonin.

Interestingly, no subsequent antidepressant can surpass the classical agents in overall efficacy in clinical trials. However, the newer agents are far safer and better tolerated.

This chapter covers the two classical antidepressants known as the MAO inhibitors and the tricyclic antidepressants. These agents dominated the treatment of depression for almost 30 years, from the late 1950s until the late 1980s when the serotonin selective reuptake inhibitors were introduced.

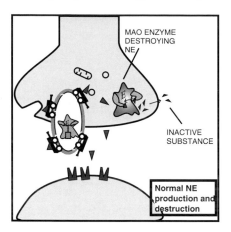

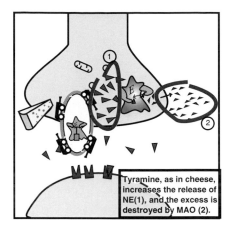

FIGURE 4.1. This figure shows the normal process of norepinephrine (noradrenaline) (NE) being both produced and destroyed. MAO (monoamine oxidase) is the enzyme which normally acts to destroy NE to keep it in balance.

FIGURE 4.2. Tyramine is an amine which is present in food, such as cheese, and wine. Indicated in this figure is how tyramine (depicted as cheese) acts to increase the release of norepinephrine (NE) (see red circle 1). However, in normal circumstances, the enzyme MAO (monoamine oxidase) readily destroys the excess NE which is released by tyramine, and no harm is done (see red circle 2).

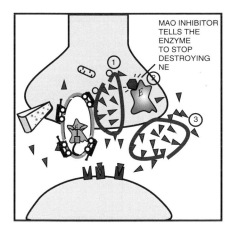

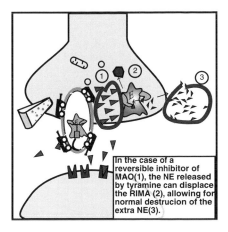

FIGURE 4.3. Actions of an irreversible and nonselective classical MAO inhibitor with tyramine.

FIGURE 4.4. Actions of a reversible inhibitor of MAO A (also known as a RIMA) with tyramine.

Here, tyramine is releasing norepinephrine (NE) (see red circle 1) just as previously shown in Figure 4.2). However, this time MAO (monoamine oxidase) is also being inhibited by a typical, irreversible MAO (monoamine oxidase) inhibitor. This results in MAO stopping its destruction of norepinephrine (NE) (see 2).

As already indicated earlier in Figure 2.9, such MAO inhibition in itself causes the accumulation of NE, and an antidepressant effect. However, when MAO inhibition is taking place in the presence of tyramine, the combination can lead to a very large accumulation of NE (see red circle 3). Such a great degree of NE accumulation can cause dangerous elevations of blood pressure.

Shown in this figure is also the combination of an MAO (monoamine oxidase) inhibitor and tyramine. However, in this case the MAO inhibitor is of the reversible type (reversible inhibitor of MAO A or RIMA). In contrast to the situation shown in the previous figure (Figure 4.3), the accumulation of norepinephrine (NE) caused by tyramine (indicated in red circle 1) can actually strip the RIMA off MAO (2). MAO - now devoid of its inhibitor - can merrily do its job, which is to destroy the NE (red circle 3) and thus prevent the dangerous accumulation of NE. Such a reversal of MAO by NE is only possible with a RIMA, and not with the classical MAO inhibitors which are completely irreversible.

Table 4.1
TYPES OF MONOAMINE OXIDASE INHIBITORS (MAOI)

CLASSICAL MAO INHIBITORS – IRREVERSIBLE AND NONSELECTIVE
   phenelzine
   tranylcypromine
   isocarboxazid
 	
RIMAs – REVERSIBLE INHIBITORS OF MAO A
   moclobemide
 	
SELECTIVE INHIBITORS OF MAO B
   deprenyl

Table 4.2
Preferred uses of classical MAO inhibitors
(NONSELECTIVE MAO A AND B IRREVERSIBLE ENZYME INHIBITION) • second line use • atypical depression (i.e., weight gain, hypersomnia, mood reactivity) • refractory cases • compliant cases • associated panic attacks

TABLE 4.1.   This lists both the classical MAO inhibitors which are nonselective and irreversible, and the newer MAO inhibitors which are selective for MAO A or MAO B and which are reversible for MAO A.

Several other RIMAs are in development, but only moclobemide is marketed (not in the US).

Tables 4.2–4.5 provide clinical tips on the modern uses of classical MAO inhibitors.

Table 4.3
Side effect profile of classical MAO inhibitors
• orthostatic hypotension • insomnia • sexual dysfunction • dietary restrictions • drug interactions/restrictions

Table 4.4
Least preferred uses of classical MAO inhibitors
• noncompliant patients • patients not highly motivated to monitor diet and concomitant medications • first line insomniac, agitated patients

Table 4.5
Clinical pearls about classical MAO inhibitors

- phenylcyclopropylamine has stimulant, amphetamine-like properties:
- insomnia managed with trazodone
- orthostatic hypotension dose related
- with great skill, can be combined in heroic cases with TCAs but never with SSRIs
- even MAO B inhibition by deprenyl is dangerous to combine with an SSRI
- reversible MAOIs specific for A can be better tolerated, fewer dietary problems, but sometimes less effective

Table 4.6
Types of tricyclic antidepressants

- clomipramine
- imipramine
- amitriptyline
- nortriptyline
- protriptyline
- maprotiline
- amoxapine
- doxepin
- desipramine
- trimipramine

This table lists many of the marketed tricyclic antidepressants. Not all are available in every country.

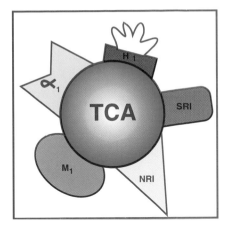

FIGURE 4.5.   Shown here is an icon of a tricyclic antidepressant (TCA). These drugs are actually five drugs in one: (1) a serotonin reuptake inhibitor (SRI); (2) a norepinephrine reuptake inhibitor (NRI); (3) an anticholinergic-antimuscarinic drug (M1); (4) an alpha 1 adrenergic antagonist (alpha 1); and (5) an antihistamine (H1).

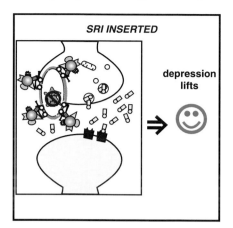

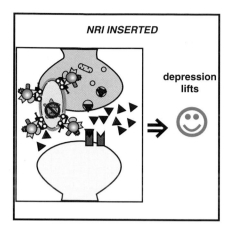

FIGURE 4.6.   Therapeutic actions of the tricyclic antidepressants (TCAs)—part 1. In this diagram, the icon of the TCA is shown with its serotonin reuptake inhibitor (SRI) portion inserted into the serotonin reuptake pump, blocking it, and causing an antidepressant effect.

FIGURE 4.7.   Therapeutic actions of the tricyclic antidepressants (TCAs)—part 2. In this diagram, the icon of the TCA is shown with its norepinephrine reuptake inhibitor (NRI) portion inserted into the norepinephrine reuptake pump, blocking it and causing an antidepressant effect. Thus, both the serotonin reuptake portion (see Figure 4.6) and the NRI portion of the TCAs act pharmacologically to cause an antidepressant effect.

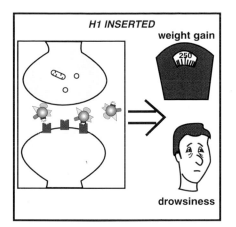

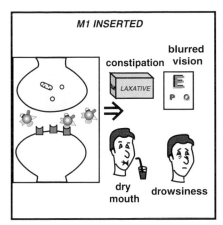

FIGURE 4.8. Side effects of the tricyclic antidepressants—part 1. The icon of the TCA is shown with its H1 (antihistamine) portion inserted into histamine receptors, causing the side effects of weight gain and drowsiness.

FIGURE 4.9. Side effects of the tricyclic antidepressants—part 2. The icon of the TCA is shown with its M1 (anticholinergic/antimuscarinic) portion inserted into acetylcholine receptors, causing the side effects of constipation, blurred vision, dry mouth and drowsiness.

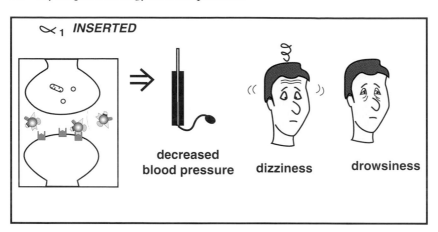

FIGURE 4.10. Side effects of the tricyclic antidepressants—part 3. On this diagram, the icon of the TCA is shown with its alpha 1 (alpha 1 adrenergic antagonist) portion inserted into alpha 1 adrenergic receptors, causing the side effects of dizziness, decreased blood pressure and drowsiness.

Tables 4.7–4.12 provide clinical tips on the modern use of classical tricyclic antidepressants.

Table 4.7

RATIONAL EXPLANATIONS FOR TRICYCLIC ANTIDEPRESSANT THERAPEUTIC EFFECTS:

Pharmacology of dual 5HT/NE uptake blockage limited by associated side-effect pharmacology

Table 4.8

RATIONAL EXPLANATIONS FOR TRICYCLIC ANTIDEPRESSANT SIDE EFFECTS

UNWANTED PHARMACOLOGIC ACTIONS AT SECONDARY RECEPTORS

Table 4.9

PREFERRED USES OF TRICYCLIC ANTIDEPRESSANTS

WELL-FITTING NICHE
• pain
• fibromyalgia
• migraine
• sedative/hypnotic
• severe depression

Table 4.10

SIDE EFFECT PROFILE OF TRICYCLIC ANTIDEPRESSANTS

• dry mouth
• blurred vision
• constipation
• urinary retention
• sedation
• orthostatic hypotension
• dizziness
• weight gain
• toxic in overdose
• confusion (especially in the elderly)

Table 4.11

LEAST PREFERRED USES OF TRICYCLIC ANTIDEPRESSANTS

• those who cannot tolerate daytime sedation, urinary retention, constipation
• overweight patients
• suicidal patients (TCAs toxic in overdose)
• cardiac illness
• multiple concomitant medications (TCA drug interactions)
• patients with dementia

Table 4.12

CLINICAL PEARLS ABOUT
TRICYCLIC ANTIDEPRESSANTS

- inexpensive
- just as effective as modern
  antidepressants
- possibly more effective in severe
  depression
- maprotiline: increased seizures;
  norepinephrine selective
- amoxapine: neuroleptic properties;
  5HT2 antagonist
- desipramine: norepinephrine
  selective
- clomipramine: most potent 5HT
  reuptake blocker of theTCAs;
  potent NE, too; effective in
  obsessive compulsive disorder;
  increased seizures at high doses

CHAPTER 5

THE SEROTONIN SELECTIVE REUPTAKE INHIBITORS

This chapter covers the serotonin selective reuptake inhibitors (SSRIs), among the most widely prescribed antidepressants throughout the world.

Five separate agents form the members of the SSRI class, differing in chemical structure, secondary pharmacologic properties and pharmacokinetics. These agents are listed in Table 5.1.

Table 5.1
There are five different SSRIs on the market in most major countries.

Serotonin selective re-uptake inhibitors (SSRIs)

- Fluoxetine
- Sertraline
- Paroxetine
- Fluvoxamine
- Citalopram

The SSRIs have revolutionized the treatment of depression for a number of reasons. The principal advantage of these drugs over the classical MAO inhibitors and tricyclic antidepressants is their much improved safety and tolerability. Whereas the classical antidepressant agents are lethal in overdose, the SSRIs are not. Also, the cardiac toxicity and troublesome anticholinergic side effects are absent from the SSRIs. This improved tolerability profile arrived on the scene just as new data demonstrated the value of long term treatment in preventing relapse of future depressive episodes. Thus, the acceptability of long term treatment is much greater with the SSRIs than with the tricyclic antidepressants, and compliance is much higher.

Another advantage of the SSRIs is the breadth of their therapeutic profile, extending far beyond antidepressant actions. Thus, SSRIs have proven efficacy in panic disorder, obsessive compulsive disorder, and bulimia with encouraging findings in social phobia, post-traumatic stress disorder, pre-menstrual dysphoric disorder, migraine, dysthymia, and many other conditions.

However, the SSRIs are not without their problems. Although efficacy is quite broad, there is a nagging feeling among many investigators that SSRIs are not as effective for severe depression as other agents with dual mechanisms such as tricyclic antidepressants, venlafaxine or mirtazapine. Also, the SSRIs do have side effects which are bothersome if not lethal. A particularly troublesome problem is the development of sexual dysfunction in long term treatment. Some of the newer agents improve on certain SSRI side effects, specifically with less anxiety, sleep disturbance and sexual dysfunction. These other agents will be discussed in the next chapter.

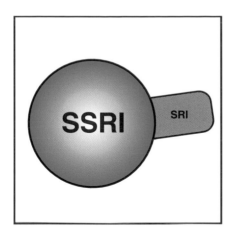

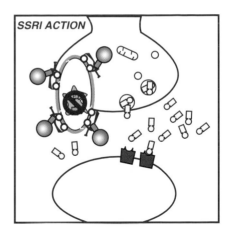

FIGURE 5.1.   Shown here is the icon of a selective serotonin reuptake inhibitor (SSRI). In this case, four out of the five pharmacological properties of the TCAs (tricyclic antidepressants; Figure 4.5) were removed. Only the serotonin reuptake inhibitor (SRI) portion remains; thus the SRI action is selective, which is why these agents are called selective SRIs.

FIGURE 5.2.   In this diagram, the SRI (serotonin reuptake inhibitor) portion of the SSRI molecule is shown inserted in the serotonin reuptake pump, blocking it and causing an antidepressant effect. This is analogous to one of the dimensions of the tricyclic antidepressants (TCAs), already shown in Figure 4.6.

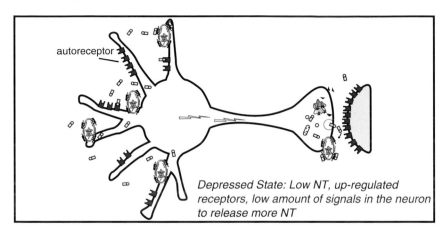

autoreceptor

Depressed State: Low NT, up-regulated receptors, low amount of signals in the neuron to release more NT

FIGURE 5.3.   Mechanism of action of serotonin selective reuptake inhibitors (SSRIs)—part 1. Depicted here is a serotonin neuron in a depressed patient. In depression, the serotonin neuron is conceptualized as having a relative deficiency of the neurotransmitter (NT) serotonin. Also, the number of serotonin receptors is upregulated, or increased, including both presynaptic autoreceptors as well as postsynaptic receptors.

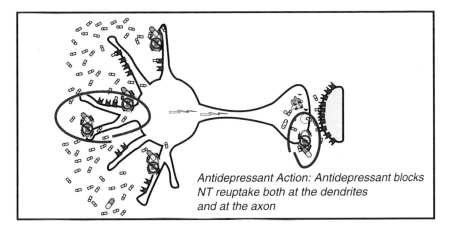

Antidepressant Action: Antidepressant blocks NT reuptake both at the dendrites and at the axon

FIGURE 5.4. Mechanism of action of serotonin selective reuptake inhibitors (SSRIs)—part 2. When an SSRI is administered, it immediately blocks the serotonin reuptake pump (see icon of a capsule blocking the reuptake pump). However, this causes the neurotransmitter (NT) serotonin to increase initially only in the somatodendritic area, and not in the axon terminals (red circle).

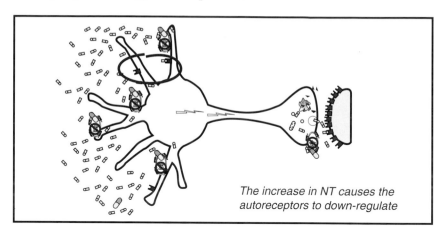

The increase in NT causes the autoreceptors to down-regulate

FIGURE 5.5.   Mechanism of action of serotonin selective reuptake inhibitors (SSRIs)—part 3. The consequence of the neurotransmitter (NT) serotonin increasing in the somatodendritic area of the serotonin neuron as depicted in Figure 5.4 is for the somatodendritic 5HT1A autoreceptors to down regulate (red circle).

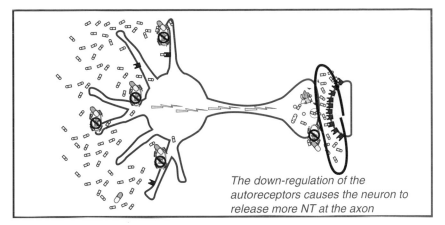

The down-regulation of the autoreceptors causes the neuron to release more NT at the axon

FIGURE 5.6.   Mechanism of action of serotonin selective reuptake inhibitors (SSRIs)—part 4. Once the somatodendritic autoreceptors down regulate as depicted in the previous figure (Fig. 5.5), there is no longer inhibition of impulse flow in the serotonin neuron. Thus, neuronal impulse flow is turned on. The consequence of this is for serotonin to be released in the axon terminal (red circle). However, this increase is delayed compared to the increase of serotonin in the somatodendritic areas of the serotonin neuron depicted earlier in Figure 5.4. This delay is the result of the time it takes for somatodendritic serotonin to down regulate the serotonin 1A autoreceptors, and turn on neuronal impulse flow in the serotonin neuron. This delay may account for why antidepressants do not relieve depression immediately. It is also the reason why the mechanism of action of antidepressants may be linked to increasing neuronal impulse flow in serotonin neurons with serotonin levels increasing in axon terminals before an SSRI can exert its antidepressant effects.

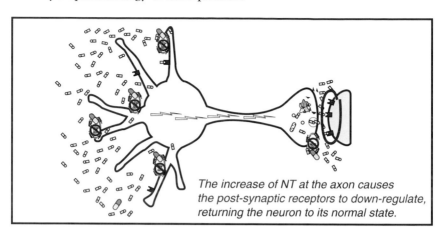

The increase of NT at the axon causes the post-synaptic receptors to down-regulate, returning the neuron to its normal state.

FIGURE 5.7.   Mechanism of action of serotonin selective reuptake inhibitors (SSRIs)—part 5. Finally, once the SSRIs have blocked the reuptake pump (Figure 5.4), increased somatodendritic serotonin (Figure 5.4), down regulated somatodendritic 5HT1A autoreceptors (Figure 5.5), turned on neuronal impulse flow (Figure 5.6) and increased release of the neurotransmitter (NT) serotonin from axon terminals (Figure 5.6), the final step shown here may be the down regulation of postsynaptic serotonin receptors. This has also been shown in previous figures demonstrating the actions of MAO (monoamine oxidase) inhibitors (Figure 2.10) and the actions of tricyclic antidepressants (Figure 2.12).

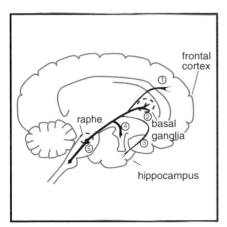

FIGURE 5.8.   Key serotonin pathways in the central nervous system. When the serotonin neuron is disinhibited, it turns on serotonin release in several pathways simultaneously. At least four of these pathways may serve as the substrate for the wide-ranging therapeutic effects of the SSRIs. Several pathways also mediate the side effect profile of the SSRIs. *Pathway 1* is from midbrain raphe to prefrontal cortex. *Pathway 2* is from midbrain raphe to basal ganglia. *Pathway 3* is from midbrain raphe to limbic cortex and hippocampus. *Pathway 4* is from midbrain raphe to hypothalamus. *Pathway 5* is from midbrain raphe descending down the spinal cord.

Table 5.2

SSRIs pharmacological profile: Serotonin's general therapeutic profile

- The pharmacology of powerful 5HT disinhibition in four key pathways

---

Table 5.3

Possible explanations for SSRI therapeutic effects: Desired 5HT1A receptor actions causing disinhibition of serotonin in theory in four key pathways

- Depression: disinhibition of the pathway to prefrontal cortex
- Obsessive compulsive disorder: disinhibition of the pathway to basal ganglia
- Panic disorder: disinhibition of the pathway to limbic cortex and hippocampus
- Bulimia: disinhibition of the pathway to hypothalamus

TABLES 5.2 and 5.3.   Clinical explanations of SSRI neurophysiology.

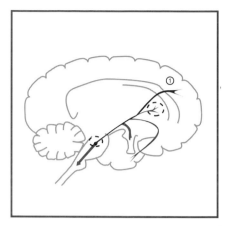

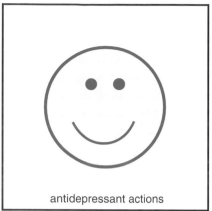

antidepressant actions

FIGURE 5.9. Antidepressant actions of the SSRIs are hypothesized to be mediated by disinhibition of serotonin in pathway 1 from midbrain raphe to prefrontal cortex. This disinhibition theoretically restores the depleted neurotransmitter in order to effect an antidepressant response, as discussed previously in chapter 2.

Table 5.4
SSRIs antidepressant profile
• Usual maintenance dose is the starting dose • Usual onset of response is 3 to 8 weeks • Target symptoms do not worsen at first • Usual response is a complete response

TABLE 5.4. Clinical tips on what to expect when using SSRIs to treat depression.

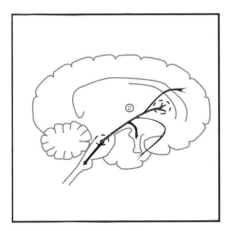

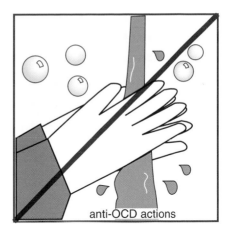

anti-OCD actions

FIGURE 5.10. Anti-obsessive compulsive disorder (OCD) actions of the SSRIs are hypothesized to be mediated by disinhibition of serotonin in pathway 2 from midbrain raphe to the basal ganglia. This disinhibition theoretically affects various pathways which use the basal ganglia as a relay station. However, there is no evidence that the SSRIs restore the depleted neurotransmitter; rather, the increase in serotonin seems to compensate for other unknown neurochemical abnormalities which may underlie the pathophysiology of OCD.

Table 5.5
SSRIs anti-OCD profile
• Usual maintenance dose is higher than the starting dose
• Usual onset of response is 12 to 26 weeks
• Target symptoms do not worsen at first
• Usual response is <50% improvement

TABLE 5.5. Clinical tips on what to expect when using SSRIs to treat obsessive compulsive disorder.

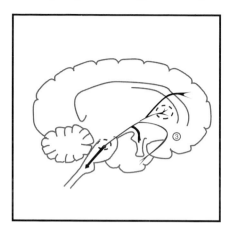

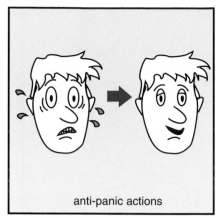

anti-panic actions

FIGURE 5.11. Anti-panic actions of the SSRIs are hypothesized to be mediated by disinhibition of serotonin in pathway 3 from midbrain raphe to the hippocampus and limbic cortex. This disinhibition theoretically activates serotonin receptors which can worsen panic or induce anxiety at first. However, after time passes, adaptations in this pathway eventually mediate antipanic actions. (See Figure 3.21 and Table 3.3. See also Table 5.9 and Figure 5.14).

Table 5.6

SSRIs anti-panic profile

- Usual starting dose is less than the starting dose for other indications
- Maintenance dose may eventually be higher than the starting dose
- Target symptoms may worsen at first
- Usual response is >50% improvement, especially in combination with other treatments such as benzodiazepines

TABLE 5.6. Clinical tips on what to expect when using SSRIs to treat panic.

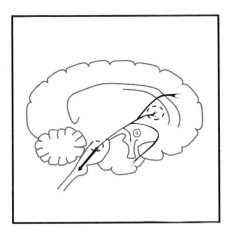 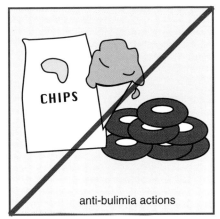

anti-bulimia actions

FIGURE 5.12.   Anti-bulimia actions of the SSRIs are hypothesized to be mediated by disinhibition of serotonin in pathway 4 from midbrain raphe to the hypothalamus. This disinhibition theoretically activates serotonin receptors which can diminish appetite and feeding behaviors.

Table 5.7

SSRIs anti-bulimia profile

- Usual starting dose is higher than the starting dose for other indications
- Maintenance dose may eventually be higher than the starting dose
- Usual onset of response may be faster than the typical antidepressant response onset of 3–8 weeks
- Target symptoms do not worsen at first
- Effectiveness in preventing relapse in acute responders is not yet established

TABLE 5.7.   Clinical tips on what to expect when using SSRIs to treat eating disorders such as bulimia and binge eating disorder.

Table 5.8
SEROTONIN SIDE EFFECT
PROFILE – pharmacology of 5HT
acting at unwanted 5HT receptors
in undesired places

- Agitation
- Akathisia
- Anxiety
- Panic attacks
- Insomnia
- Sexual dysfunction
    Lack of desire from
    decreasing dopamine in meso-
    limbic pleasure centres
    Lack of orgasm or ejaculation
    from inhibiting spinal reflexes
- Nausea
- GI distress/diarrhoea
- Headache
- Withdrawal effects
- Long term wearing off of efficacy

Table 5.9
Side effect profile of an SSRI:
consequences of stimulating 5HT2
receptors.

WHEN SSRIs STIMULATE 5HT2
RECEPTORS

- Agitation
- Akathisia
- Anxiety
- Panic attacks
- Insomnia
- Sexual dysfunction

Table 5.10
Side effect profile of an SSRI:
consequences of stimulating 5HT3
receptors

WHEN SSRIs STIMULATE 5HT3
RECEPTORS

- Nausea
- Gastrointestinal (GI) distress
- Diarrhoea
- Headache

TABLES 5.8–5.10 provide clinical
explanations for the side effects of the
SSRIs.

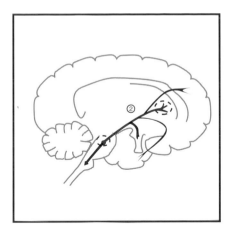
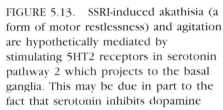

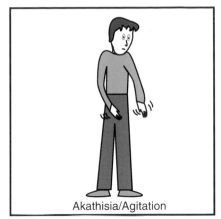

Akathisia/Agitation

FIGURE 5.13.   SSRI-induced akathisia (a form of motor restlessness) and agitation are hypothetically mediated by stimulating 5HT2 receptors in serotonin pathway 2 which projects to the basal ganglia. This may be due in part to the fact that serotonin inhibits dopamine release there. Thus, increasing serotonin can produce a mild pseudo-dopamine deficiency state and the concomitant symptoms of akathisia and agitation. Overt extrapyramidal effects can even be caused in rare cases.

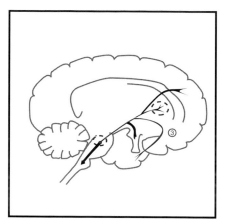 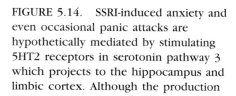

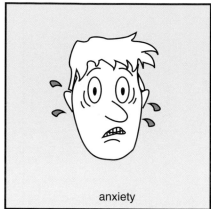

anxiety

FIGURE 5.14. SSRI-induced anxiety and even occasional panic attacks are hypothetically mediated by stimulating 5HT2 receptors in serotonin pathway 3 which projects to the hippocampus and limbic cortex. Although the production of anxiety is often seen at the initiation of treatment with an SSRI, it usually subsides over time and the SSRIs eventually are long-term anxiolytics.

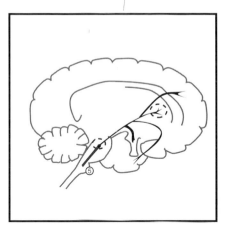

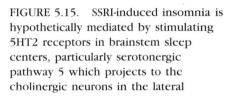

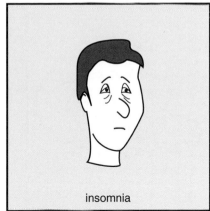

FIGURE 5.15.   SSRI-induced insomnia is hypothetically mediated by stimulating 5HT2 receptors in brainstem sleep centers, particularly serotonergic pathway 5 which projects to the cholinergic neurons in the lateral tegmentum. Stimulating 5HT2 disrupts particularly slow wave sleep. This can also induce nocturnal myoclonus which can increase the frequency of nocturnal awakenings.

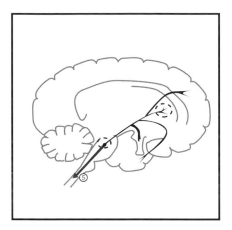 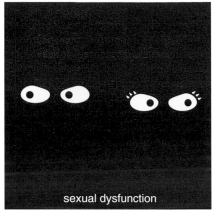

sexual dysfunction

FIGURE 5.16. SSRI-induced sexual dysfunction. Sexual function has a complex physiology and psychology. Some forms of sexual dysfunction can be caused by the illnesses which SSRIs treat, especially depression. This usually takes the form of decreased libido and reduced pleasurability, leading even to reduction in arousal. These aspects of sexual functioning may be mediated by mesolimbic dopamine pathways. This pathway, which may be inhibited by serotonergic input to 5HT2 receptors, is hypothesized to control pleasure and reward. Abnormalities in this pathway may be associated with conditions such as anhedonia in depression, and craving from withdrawal of substances of abuse.

Simply put, there is a reciprocal relationship between serotonin and dopamine, with serotonin tending to inhibit sexual functioning and dopamine tending to enhance sexual functioning. That is why the SSRIs, which disinhibit serotonergic pathways innervating mesolimbic dopamine systems, can cause sexual dysfunction. This is also why agents which promote dopamine, such as stimulants, can often reverse SSRI-induced sexual dysfunction.

Another key serotonin pathway which controls sexual function is the descending pathway from brainstem down the spinal cord to spinal neurons mediating various spinal reflexes such as ejaculation and orgasm (pathway 5). Disinhibiting this descending spinal pathway for serotonin causes increased serotonin release which in turn inhibits sexual functioning.

Evidence for serotonin mediating its negative effects on sexual functioning via 5HT2 receptors comes both from observations that 5HT2 antagonists can occasionally reverse SSRI-induced sexual dysfunction. Also, those antidepressants which are 5HT2 antagonists do not seem to induce sexual dysfunction.

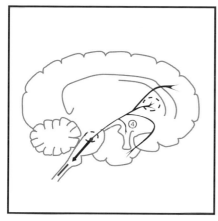

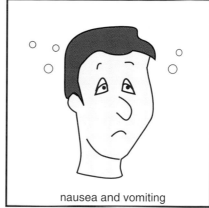

nausea and vomiting

FIGURE 5.17.   The brainstem vomiting center, also known as the chemoreceptor trigger zone, can be triggered by 5HT3 agonists, such as serotonin itself, or even cancer chemotherapy. Blocking this receptor can prevent cancer chemotherapy from inducing vomiting.

Disinhibition of serotonin pathway 4 from brainstem to hypothalamus which mediates aspects of appetite and eating behaviors may be responsible for the reduced appetite, nausea and even weight loss associated with SSRIs.

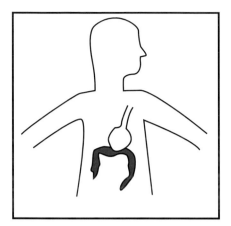

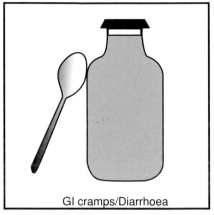

GI cramps/Diarrhoea

FIGURE 5.18. Finally, there are 5HT3 receptors located right in the wall of the gut, which when stimulated increase GI motility. Thus, increases in serotonin in the gut which are induced by SSRIs may be responsible for the GI cramps and diarrhoea associated with SSRI administration.

TABLES 5.11–5.17 provide clinical tips on how to use, and what to expect from using, SSRIs, based on art and anecdote as well as on science.

Table 5.11
Clinical Pearls about SSRIs

- Different doses, different onsets of action, different tolerabilities and different degrees of efficacy in various therapeutic targets
- Most side effects short term, and immediate, with tolerance developing
- Different tolerability and efficacy profiles for individual patients treated by different agents within the class
- Concomitant agents often boost efficacy and/or enhance tolerability
- Less efficacy than TCAs for severe depression?
- Wearing off of efficacy over long treatment intervals?
- For sexual dysfunction, switch to nefazodone, mirtazapine or bupropion.
- For sexual dysfunction add serotonergic agents: cyproheptadine, nefazodone or buspirone
- For sexual dysfunction add dopaminergic agents: amantadine, bromocriptine, methylphenidate, d-amphetamine

Table 5.12
Fluoxetine Pearls

- Consider for atypical depression
- Consider avoiding for agitated insomniacs who wish to avoid sexual dysfunction
- FDA label for depression, OCD and (almost) for bulimia
- Not as well tolerated without co-therapy for panic
- Long half life; even longer lasting active metabolite
- Less selective over norepinephrine and 5HT2C
- Inhibits 2D6

Table 5.13
Sertraline Pearls

- Weak 2D6 inhibitor
- More diarrhoea
- FDA label for depression and OCD
- Often activating and panicogenic in panic disorder
- Least selective over dopamine
- Consider for atypical depression
- Consider avoiding in patients with multiple GI somatic symptoms, agitation and/or insomnia who wish to avoid sexual dysfunction

Table 5.14
Paroxetine Pearls

- Potent 2D6 inhibitor
- NOT linear dosing (i.e., 20, 30, 40 mg)
- Inhibits own metabolism
- Least selective over acetylcholine, thus some mild anticholinergic side effects
- FDA label in USA for depression, panic and OCD
- Washout can be too rapid with withdrawal effects, especially movement disorders, akathisia, dystonia, restlessness, and GI symptoms plus dizziness
- Generally well tolerated in panic
- Consider for mixed anxiety depression
- Consider avoiding in patients with hypersomnia, retardation, insomniacs or those who wish to avoid sexual dysfunction.

Table 5.15
Fluvoxamine Pearls

- Consider for mixed anxiety depression
- FDA label for OCD, approved in Europe for depression, generally well tolerated and effective in panic
- May have a lower incidence of sexual dysfunction than other SSRIs
- Blocks metabolism of theophylin so reduce theophylin dose if given concomitantly
- Some withdrawal effects, GI side effects
- Consider avoiding in patients with multiple GI somatic complaints, agitation, and/or insomnia who wish to avoid sexual dysfunction

Table 5.17
Least preferred uses of SSRIs

- Sexual dysfunction
- Major relationship problems where the development of sexual dysfunction could be problematic
- Secondary refractoriness (i.e. loss of efficacy with long term treatment)
- When nocturnal myoclonus is present
- Patients with consistent insomnia and agitation

Table 5.16
Citalopram Pearls

- Most selective SSRI
- Weak inhibitor of 2D6
- Safety in overdose?
- FDA approval pending
- Consider avoiding in patients with agitation and sleep disturbance
- Less sexual dysfunction?

CHAPTER 6

OTHER NEUROTRANSMITTER MECHANISMS

In this chapter, several new classes of antidepressants are presented, all working on neurotransmitter mechanisms different from the SSRIs. They all act differently to the classical monoamine oxidase inhibitors and tricyclic antidepressants.

These agents are venlafaxine, trazodone, nefazodone, mianserin (not available in the US), mirtazapine and bupropion.

ANTIDEPRESSANTS ACTING BY OTHER NEUROTRANSMITTER MECHANISMS

- venlafaxine
  serotonin and norepinephrine (and possibly dopamine) reuptake
  blockades
- trazodone
  serotonin 2 antagonism and serotonin reuptake blockade with strong
  alpha 1 antagonism and antihistamine properties
- nefazodone
  serotonin 2 antagonism and serotonin and norepinephrine reuptake
  blockades
- mianserin
  alpha 2 antagonist with potent alpha 1, serotonin 2 and histamine 1
  antagonist properties
- mirtazapine
  NaSSA (Noradrenergic and Specific Serotonergic Antidepressant
  alpha 2 antagonist with potent serotonin 2, serotonin 3 and histamine 1
  antagonist properties
- bupropion
  norepinephrine and dopamine reuptake inhibitor

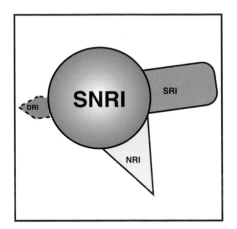

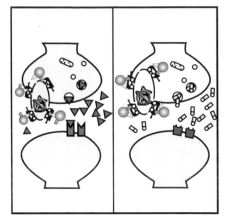

FIGURE 6.1.   Shown here is the icon of a dual reuptake inhibitor which combines the actions of both a serotonin reuptake inhibitor (SRI) and a norepinephrine reuptake inhibitor (NRI). At very high doses there is even a bit of dopamine reuptake blockade (DRI). This agent is venlafaxine.

For this agent, 3 out of the 5 pharmacological properties of the TCAs (tricyclic antidepressants; Figure 4.5) were removed. Both the SRI portion and the NRI portion of the TCA remain; however the alpha, antihistamine and anticholinergic portions are removed.

Venlafaxine is considered to be a serotonin/norepinephrine reuptake inhibitor an SNRI or dual reuptake inhibitor from a pharmacological point of view.

FIGURE 6.2.   In this diagram, the dual actions of the serotonin/norepinephrine reuptake inhibitor (SNRI) venlafaxine is shown. Both the NRI (norepinephrine reuptake inhibitor) portion of the SNRI molecule (left panel) and the SRI (serotonin reuptake inhibitor) portion of the SNRI molecule (right panel) are inserted into their respective reuptake pumps. Consequently, both reuptake pumps are blocked, and the drug mediates an antidepressant effect. This is analogous to two of the dimensions of the tricyclic antidepressants (TCAs), already shown in Figure 4.6 and 4.7.

TABLES 6.1–6.7 provide clinical tips on how to use venlafaxine and what to expect from using venlafaxine based on art and anecdotes as well as science.

Table 6.1

PHARMACOLOGICAL PROFILE OF VENLAFAXINE:

- the pharmacology of 1, 2 or all 3 monoamines, depending upon dose
- at low doses only serotonin reuptake blockade
- at medium to high doses, both serotonin and norepinephrine reuptake blockade
- at very high doses, three monoamine reuptakes blocked: namely dopamine as well as serotonin and norepinephrine

---

Table 6.2

THERAPEUTIC PROFILE OF VENLAFAXINE:

- at medium to high doses, use for melancholic, severely depressed, inpatients and those refractory to other antidepressants
- at low doses no reason to think of this drug any differently than as an SSRI
- use in retarded, hypersomnic, weight gaining, atypical depressives

---

Table 6.3

PHARMACOLOGY OF VENLAFAXINE SIDE EFFECTS

- low dose pharmacology, same as SSRIs
- intermediate to high doses mediated by additional proadrenergic actions

---

Table 6.4

VENLAFAXINE SIDE EFFECTS AT LOW DOSES: (SAME AS SSRIs)

- nausea
- agitation
- sexual dysfunction
- insomnia

Table 6.5

VENLAFAXINE SIDE EFFECTS AT MEDIUM TO HIGH DOSES: (MEDIATED BY NOREPIN-EPHRINE AND DOPAMINE AS WELL AS SEROTONIN)

- hypertension
- severe insomnia
- severe agitation
- severe nausea
- headache

Table 6.6

CLINICAL PEARLS ABOUT VENLAFAXINE

- three drugs in one:
  - SSRI at low doses (essentially a twice a day SSRI)
  - add NE uptake blockade at medium to high doses
  - add DA reuptake at high to very high doses
- choose the dose, and therefore choose which drug you want
- no advantage over SSRI at low doses
- possibly more rapid in onset of action than other antidepressants
- possibly useful at medium to very high doses for cases refractory to SSRIs
- not well tolerated at medium to high doses
- zolpidem or trazodone may be useful for venlafaxine's insomnia
- mirtazapine may be useful for venlafaxine's nausea, insomnia and agitation
- venlafaxine withdrawal effects common (GI, dizziness, sweating, etc);
- controlled release formulation in testing for once a day use; until then use twice daily dosing
- low likelihood of drug interactions (other than MAOIs)

Table 6.7

LEAST PREFERRED USES FOR VENLAFAXINE

- agitated
- anxious
- panicky
- insomniac
- weight loss
- sexual dysfunction
- noncompliance with twice daily dosing
- patients who have trouble following an up-titration program arriving at optimal dosing
- borderline or labile hypertension

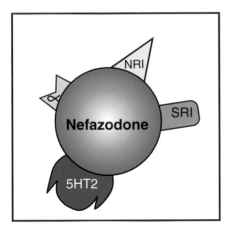

FIGURE 6.3.   Shown here is the icon for the 5HT2 antagonist, nefazodone. Several psychotropic agents share the property of blocking 5HT2 receptors in addition to nefazodone. It is important not to lump these agents together because all available 5HT2 antagonists have additional important pharmacological properties. These other actions distinguish one agent from another in a manner important for a prescriber of these agents to understand. For nefazodone, its most powerful action of 5HT2 receptor blockade is coupled with less powerful serotonin reuptake blockade.

Table 6.8

SEROTONIN 2 ANTAGONISTS IN PSYCHIATRIC PRACTICE ALL HAVE ADDITIONAL IMPORTANT PHARMACOLOGIC ACTIONS

- nefazodone (also SRI)
- trazodone (no NRI; blocks histamine receptors)
- several tricyclic antidepressants (e.g., amoxapine; amitriptyline; nortriptyline) (see Figures 4.6–4.10)
- cyproheptadine (used predominantly as an antihistamine)
- clozapine (the classical atypical antipsychotic)
- methysergide (used to treat migraine)
- new atypical antipsychotics (e.g., risperidone, olanzapine)
- mianserin (also alpha 1 and 2)
- mirtazapine (NaSSA, see Figures 6.6–6.15)

Table 6.9

CLINICALLY IMPORTANT CONSEQUENCES OF BLOCKING 5HT2 RECEPTORS

- Reduce anxiety
- Enhance slow wave sleep
- Causes no sexual dysfunction
- Sedation

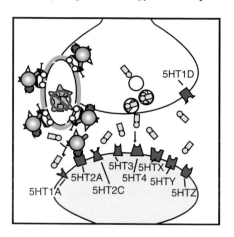

FIGURE 6.4.   Nefazodone is a serotonin antagonist and a reuptake inhibitor (SARI). It acts by potent blockade both of 5HT2 receptors (see postsynaptic 5HT2A receptor above), combined with lesser SRI (serotonin reuptake inhibitor) (see presynaptic 5HT reuptake pump above) and NRI (norepinephrine reuptake inhibitor) and alpha 1 antagonist actions. Nefazodone's NRI tends to counter its alpha adrenergic blocking properties so that little net alpha 1 antagonism results.

Trazodone is also a 5HT2 antagonist and a SRI, but lacks NRI properties. Trazodone also contains antihistamine properties and alpha 1 antagonist properties. These differences may account for the observation that nefazodone is a far less sedating and perhaps a more effective antidepressant than trazodone.

In this diagram, the dual actions of a serotonin 2 antagonist/reuptake inhibitor (SARI) of nefazodone are shown. Nefazodone thus acts both presynaptically and postsynaptically.

Presynaptic actions are indicated by the serotonin reuptake inhibitor (SRI) portion of the icon inserted into the serotonin reuptake pump, blocking it. Postsynaptic actions are indicated by the serotonin 2 receptor antagonist portion of the icon (5HT2) inserted into the serotonin 2 receptor, blocking it.

It is believed that both actions contribute to the therapeutic actions of nefazodone as an antidepressant. Blocking serotonin actions at 5HT2 receptors may also diminish the side effects associated with stimulating 5HT2 receptors. The serotonin 2 antagonist properties are stronger than the serotonin reuptake properties, so serotonin antagonism predominates at 5HT2 receptor (see Table 5.9 and Figures 5.13–5.16).

TABLES 6.10–6.16 provide clinical tips on how to use nefazodone, and what to expect from using nefazodone, based on art and anecdote as well as on science.

Table 6.10
PHARMACOLOGICAL PROFILE OF NEFAZODONE • powerful 5HT2 receptor antagonism plus 5HT reuptake blockade

Table 6.11

THERAPEUTIC PROFILE OF NEFAZODONE
 	
• depression in association with anxiety
  agitation
  sleep disturbance
  insomnia
• for prior SSRI-induced sexual dysfunction
• inability to tolerate SSRIs
• for SSRI responders who lose their response

Table 6.12
PHARMACOLOGY OF NEFAZODONE'S SIDE EFFECTS • some side effects due to excessive blockade of 5HT2 receptors • other side effects due to mCPP metabolite, a 5HT2A/2C agonist

Table 6.13
SIDE EFFECTS OF NEFAZODONE FROM 5HT2 BLOCKADE • somnolence • palinopsia (visual streaking; rare) • asthenia

Table 6.14

SIDE EFFECTS OF NEFAZODONE DUE TO MCPP METABOLITE FORMATION
 	
• 4% of caucasians lack the enzyme cytochrome P450 2D6
  – prior treatment with SSRIs inhibits cytochrome P450 2D6
  – if 2D6 absent or inhibited, lots of mCPP can form, leading to stimulation rather than blockade of 5HT2A/2C receptors causing the opposite effects of the parent compound nefazodone itself
• dizziness, lightheadedness
• insomnia
• agitation
• nausea (also from stimulating 5HT3 receptors)

Table 6.15
NEFAZODONE PEARLS • be careful in switching from or adding to SSRIs i.e., titrate down on the SSRI and titrate up on nefazodone or side effects will result from the drug interaction • agitation and flu-like distress upon first dosing may indicate genetic lack of 2D6 or SSRI- induced 2D6 inhibition from residual SSRI during switching, thus making more mCPP, an anxiogenic metabolite • palinopsia due to partial agonism rather than silent antagonism at 5HT2 receptors • do not underdose the elderly • patients may tolerate all dosing once daily at night • do not confuse with trazodone, which is much more sedating • for elderly patients with early dementia and agitated depression consider nefazodone qAM plus additional trazodone qhs

Table 6.16
LEAST PREFERRED USES OF NEFAZODONE • those with no 2D6 • hypersomnic, regressed, retarded depressed patient • noncompliance with bid dosing • patients who have trouble following an up-titration program arriving at optimal dosing

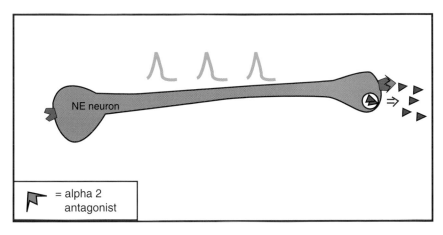

NE neuron

⬧ = alpha 2
   antagonist

FIGURE 6.5.   Mianserin was the first alpha 2 antagonist introduced as an antidepressant. Because of this property, mianserin can disinhibit noradrenergic neurons. It does this by blocking a normally inhibitory presynaptic alpha 2 autoreceptor.

Although this might also be expected to disinhibit serotonin neurons as well by blocking the alpha 2 heteroreceptors which also exist on serotonin axons, this does not seem to be the case because mianserin also blocks alpha 1 receptors. This tends to mitigate the effects of alpha 2 antagonism on serotonergic neurons.

The new agent mirtazapine retains the effects on the noradrenergic neuron, but also extends the disinhibition to serotonin neurons, since mirtazapine is more selective for alpha 2 receptors over alpha 1 receptors compared to mianserin.

Mianserin is sedating because it also has antihistamine properties. Finally, mianserin is a serotonin 2 antagonist, therefore lacking the anxiogenic, sleep disrupting and sexual dysfunction-inducing properties of the SSRIs.

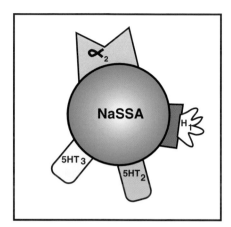

FIGURE 6.6.   Mirtazapine, a Noradrenergic and Specific Serotonergic Antidepressant (NaSSA).

Shown here is an icon for mirtazapine, the NaSSA with four principal pharmacological actions. The most important to the therapeutic effects in depression is the alpha 2 antagonist property, which acts to disinhibit both the NE and the 5HT neurons and consequently increase both NE and 5HT 1A mediated neurotransmission. The second and third properties are 5HT2 and 5HT3 antagonism, which probably are most important in improving the tolerability profile of mirtazapine compared to non-selective serotonin agents such as the SSRIs. Finally, mirtazapine has potent antihistaminergic properties, which contribute both to reducing the anxiogenic effects of increased NE, and to the side effects of weight gain and sedation.

Table 6.17
CLINICALLY IMPORTANT CONSEQUENCES OF BLOCKING ALPHA 2 RECEPTORS
• antidepressant actions • increasing NE neurotransmission • increasing 5HT neurotransmission

Table 6.18
CLINICALLY IMPORTANT CONSEQUENCES OF STIMULATING 5HT1A RECEPTORS WHILE BLOCKING 5HT2 AND 5HT3 RECEPTORS
• antidepressant actions • anxiolytic actions • sleep enhancing/restoring actions • little or no sexual dysfunction • little or no nausea or diarrhoea

MIRTAZAPINE: A DESIGNER DRUG WITH NOVEL ACTIONS KNOWN PHARMACOLOGICALLY AS NaSSA (NORADRENERGIC AND SPECIFIC SEROTONERGIC ANTIDEPRESSANT)

Mirtazapine is a 'designer' antidepressant with four principal actions which combine to make a quite novel compound. Although mirtazapine could be classified simply as an alpha 2 antagonist, this designation does not do justice to its other important pharmacological properties.

One name appropriate for mirtazapine is NaSSA, or Noradrenergic and Specific Serotonergic Antidepressant. By this, it is implied that mirtazapine enhances both noradrenergic and serotonergic neurotransmission and that its serotonergic actions are selectively directed away from the 5HT2 and 5HT3 receptors, to the 5HT1A receptor.

This is the only dual action drug which can enhance the availability of both norepinephrine and serotonin, and to do it by blocking alpha 2 receptors rather than by blocking a neurotransmitter reuptake pump. Also, mirtazapine exploits the interactions between NE and 5HT explained earlier in Figures 3.23 to 3.28 in order to attain its dual pharmacologic actions.

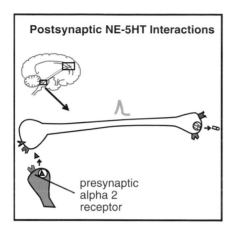

Postsynaptic NE-5HT Interactions

presynaptic
alpha 2
receptor

FIGURE 6.7.   Here the noradrenergic
neuron at the bottom is making a
postsynaptic connection with the
serotonergic neuron.

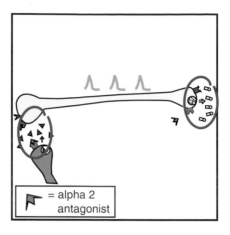

= alpha 2
antagonist

FIGURE 6.8.   When the NE neuron is
disinhibited by mirtazapine's alpha 2
antagonism (at the alpha 2 autoreceptor
on the NE neuron at the bottom) the
normal ability of NE to inhibit its own
release is gone. The result is an increase
in NE release, and NE neurotransmission,
indicated within the red circle on the left.

There is a second consequence to this
disinhibition of NE, namely that the 5HT
neuron is stimulated, causing 5HT release
as well. This is indicated within the red
circle on the right. Enhanced 5HT
neurotransmission is made possible by 2
mechanisms. Firstly, low affinity at
mirtazapine for alpha 1 receptors located
at 5HT cell bodies allows the released NE
to increase the firing rate of 5HT neurons.
This is indicated by the increased NE
within the red circle on the left driving
5HT out of the serotonin neuron
indicated by the increased 5HT within the
red circle on the right. Secondly,
mirtazapine blocks alpha 2
heteroreceptors at 5HT terminals. This is
indicated later in Figure 6.10. The net
result is an increase in 5HT release and in
5HT neurotransmission.

Figure 6.8 demonstrates how mirtazapine
increases both NE and 5HT, both of
which are the desired actions of an
effective antidepressant agent.

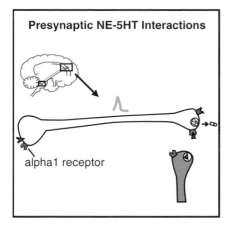

Presynaptic NE-5HT Interactions

alpha1 receptor

FIGURE 6.9.   Here the noradrenergic neuron at the bottom is making a connection with the presynaptic axon terminal of the serotonin neuron.

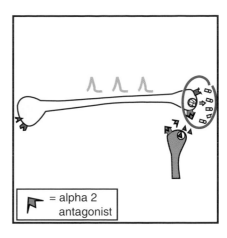

= alpha 2 antagonist

FIGURE 6.10.   Mirtazapine's alpha 2 antagonist properties block the alpha 2 heteroreceptors at 5HT terminals (shown inside the red circle). The net result is an increase in 5HT release and in 5HT neurotransmission (also shown inside the red circle).

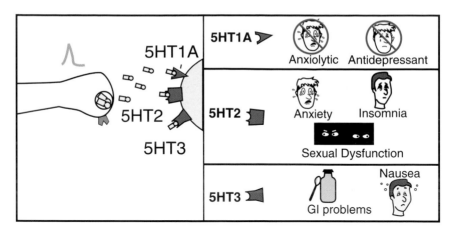

FIGURE 6.11.   The next three figures show how mirtazapine is designed to cause selective rather than indiscriminate serotonin and norepinephrine actions. Although it is desirable to increase both serotonin and norepinephrine to produce an antidepressant effect, it is not desirable to do this indiscriminately.

The figures which follow show how mirtazapine's pharmacological design counters the stimulating and anxiogenic effects of indiscriminate norepinephrine actions. They also show how other aspects of mirtazapine's pharmacological design counteract the unwanted effects of indiscriminate serotonin actions at unwanted serotonin receptors.

Shown in Figure 6.11 above is the robust disinhibition of serotonin leading to nonselective serotonin actions at all 5HT receptor subtypes. Thus, Figure 6.11 shows how there is a such thing as too much serotonin. This is seen when antidepressants increase serotonin at all receptor subtypes, thus creating the 'serotonin side effect profile' explained earlier in Tables 5.8-5.10 and Figures 5.13-5.18 for the SSRIs.

When serotonin acts at all serotonin receptor subtypes, it causes not only desired antidepressant and anxiolytic effects, but also undesired side effects such as insomnia, sexual dysfunction, and nausea. This is essentially the serotonergic profile of the SSRIs (see Figures 5.13-5.18).

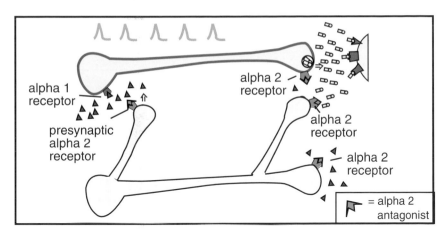

FIGURE 6.12.   If mirtazapine were a pure alpha 2 antagonist, this single action would cause disinhibition of both serotonin and norepinephrine, and this action would be fairly ubiquitous. As will be explained in the next few figures, mirtazapine is more than an alpha 2 antagonist. Nevertheless, it is the alpha 2 antagonist action of mirtazapine which results in the desired increases in both serotonin and norepinephrine (see also Table 6.17).

However, there is a such thing as too much norepinephrine and too much serotonin. Robust disinhibition of NE, for example, is associated with anxiety.

The disinhibition of the serotonin neuron is shown in the top neuron and the serotonin release to the right. Actions at both desired and undesired serotonin receptors are possible (see also Tables 5.8–5.10 and Figures 5.13 to 5.18).

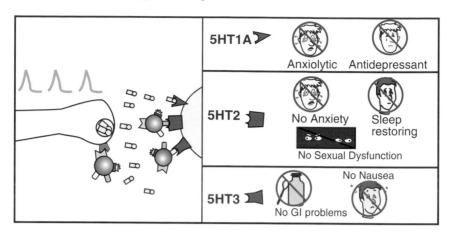

FIGURE 6.13.   In contrast to agents which increase serotonin ubiquitously at all 5HT receptors, mirtazapine is designed to direct serotonin to the 5HT1A receptor, since the 5HT2 and 5HT3 receptors are blocked. This results in retaining the favorable antidepressant therapeutic actions when serotonin is increased, yet reducing the unwanted side effects associated with stimulation of the 5HT2 and 5HT3 receptors (see also Table 6.18).

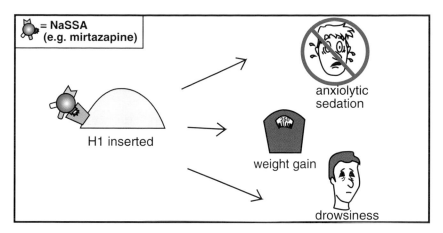

FIGURE 6.14.   Mirtazapine is endowed with antihistamine properties. This is a 'good news/bad news' pharmacologic characteristic. The 'good news' is that the antihistamine properties counteract the anxiogenic actions of indiscriminate NE release, as well as promote anxiolytic and sedative/hypnotic actions. The 'bad news' is that antihistamine properties are associated with weight gain and drowsiness.

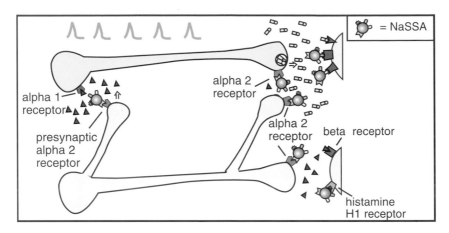

FIGURE 6.15.   This figure shows the integrated story of how mirtazapine's design produces a noradrenergic and specific serotonergic antidepressant (NaSSA).

The fundamental action is to increase both 5HT and NE via alpha 2 antagonism (Table 6.17).

Addition of antihistaminergic properties counteracts the anxiogenic effects of excessive NE.

Addition of 5HT2 and 5HT3 antagonist properties counteracts the numerous side effects of 5HT acting nonselectively at these receptors (Table 6.18).

TABLES 6.19–6.22 provide clinical tips on how to use mirtazapine and what to expect from using mirtazapine based on art and anecdote as well as science.

Table 6.19

MIRTAZAPINE THERAPEUTIC PROFILE

Depression associated with

- anxiety
- agitation
- insomnia
- SSRI-induced:
  - sexual dysfunction
  - nausea
  - GI disturbance
- panic
- weight loss
- severe depression
- for SSRI responders who have lost their response

Table 6.20

MIRTAZAPINE SIDE-EFFECT PROFILE

Predominantly the pharmacology of histamine H1 receptor antagonism

- sedation
- weight gain

Table 6.21

LEAST PREFERRED USES OF MIRTAZAPINE

- hypersomnia
- motor retardation
- cognitive slowing
- overweight

Table 6.22

CLINICAL PEARLS FOR MIRTAZAPINE

- sedation may be INVERSELY related to dose
- lowering dose may thus increase sedation
- two mechanisms (NE plus 5-HT) may be better than one (5HT alone) for severe or refractory depression
- consider for panic disorder
- consider for mixed anxiety depression
- low likelihood of drug interactions (except MAOI)
- adding alpha-2 antagonism to agents which act as reuptake blockers may be useful for refractory depression
- adding mirtazapine's 5-HT2 antagonism may reduce SSRI- or venlafaxine-induced anxiety or insomnia
- adding mirtazapine's 5-HT3 antagonism may reduce SSRI- or venlafaxine-induced nausea

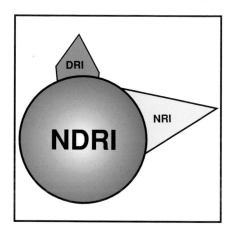

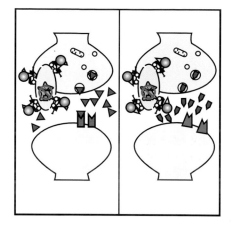

FIGURE 6.16.   Shown here is the icon of the norepinephrine and dopamine reuptake inhibitor (NDRI) known as bupropion which is only available in the USA. Bupropion is a norepinephrine reuptake inhibitor (NRI) as well as a dopamine reuptake inhibitor (DRI).

FIGURE 6.17.   In this diagram, the NRI (norepinephrine reuptake inhibitor) and the DRI (dopamine reuptake inhibitor) portions of the NDRI molecule are shown inserted in the norepinephrine and the dopamine reuptake pumps, respectively, blocking them and causing an antidepressant effect.

TABLES 6.23–6.26 provide clinical tips on how to use bupropion and what to expect from using bupropion based on art and anecdote as well as on science.

Table 6.23
BUPROPION THERAPEUTIC PROFILE
• retarded depression • hypersomnia • nonresponders to serotonergic agents • nontolerators of serotonergic agents • no sexual dysfunction • cognitive slowing/pseudodementia

Table 6.24
BUPROPION SIDE EFFECT PROFILE
• stimulating • agitation • nausea • insomnia • seizures (4/1000)

Table 6.25
LEAST PREFERRED USES FOR BUPROPION
• seizure disorder patients • seizure prone/head injury • noncompliant to multiple daily dosing • agitated, insomniac patients

Table 6.26
CLINICAL PEARLS ABOUT BUPROPION
• can add to SSRIs to reverse SSRI sexual dysfunction • can add to SSRIs to boost inadequate efficacy • can switch SSRI secondary refractory patients to reattain efficacy • new controlled release formulation for twice daily and possibly once daily administration • use in adult and childhood ADD (attention deficit disorder) • effective for use in smoking cessation (treatment of nicotine dependence) • may be useful for treating stimulant withdrawal and craving

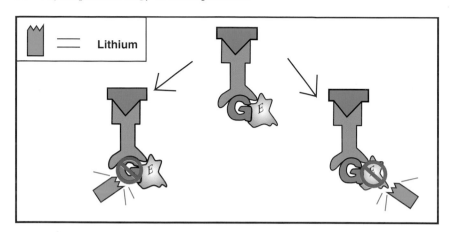

FIGURE 6.18. The mechanism of action of lithium is not well understood, but is hypothesized to act by modifying second messenger systems. One possibility is that lithium alters G-proteins and their ability to transduce signals inside the cell once the neurotransmitter receptor is occupied by the neurotransmitter. Another theory is that lithium alters enzymes which interact with the second messenger system, such as inositol monophosphatase, or others.

CHAPTER 7

ANTIDEPRESSANT SUMMARY

Chapters 4-6 have detailed the more than 24 antidepressant agents (Figure 7.1) which work by seven distinct pharmacological mechanisms (Figure 7.2). It can be a daunting task to select a particular antidepressant drug for an individual patient given this embarrassment of riches. Prescribing decisions can be made by cost considerations, safety, side effect profile, prior response to antidepressant therapy, or pure marketing considerations. Such selections are, however, not always rational.

The approach advocated here is to understand the pharmacological mechanisms of action of the various available agents, and to use this information to predict, as far as is possible, the antidepressant with a preferred tolerability and effectiveness profile for an individual patient.

Pharmacological mechanisms are better predictors of side effects than they are of antidepressant efficacy. One approach to making an individual prescribing decision, therefore, is to attempt to match patient symptom profiles to anticipated drug side effect profiles to select a likely best fit. This idea is presented here in a summary table (Table 7.1).

In terms of effectiveness, there is a growing body of evidence suggesting that drugs with two pharmacological mechanisms (i.e., acting on both serotonin and norepinephrine) may be preferred over drugs with just one action (e.g., SSRIs) for severely depressed melancholic inpatients. Combining mechanisms is the theme for managing treatment resistant cases (see Chapter 8), so it may also be preferable at times to use a single agent with multiple mechanisms for such treatment resistant cases.

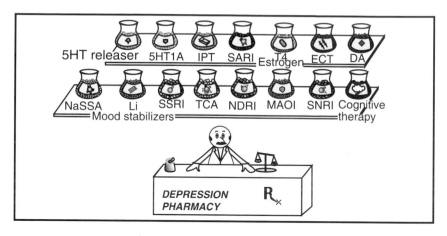

FIGURE 7.1   The modern therapeutic armamentarium for the depression pharmacy includes numerous agents working by many different mechanisms. These agents are on the shelves above and are also shown in Figure 7.2. They include TCA (tricyclic antidepressants), SSRI (serotonin selective reuptake inhibitors), NDRI (norepinephrine and dopamine reuptake inhibitor), NaSSA (noradrenergic and specific serotonergic antidepressant), SNRI (sertonin and norepinephrine reuptake inhibitor), SARI (serotonin antagonist and reuptake inhibitor) and MAOI (monoamine oxidase inhibitors). Many of these single agents have multiple mechanisms (see also Figure 7.2).

Yet other agents are used in combination with antidepressants to add a different pharmacologic mechanism and hopefully enhance the first agent's tolerability or efficacy.

Those such agents shown in the depression pharmacy above include 5HT releasers (e.g. fenfluramine), 5HT1A agents (such as bupropion or pindolol), IPT (interpersonal psychotherapy), T4 (thyroxin), estrogen, ECT (electroconvulsive therapy), DA (dopaminergic stimulants such as bromocriptine, methylphenidate and d-amphetamine), Li (lithium), mood stabilizers (various anticonvulsants such as valproic acid and carbamazepine), and cognitive psychotherapy.

The art and science of mixing these agents and their mechanism is the theme of Chapter 8.

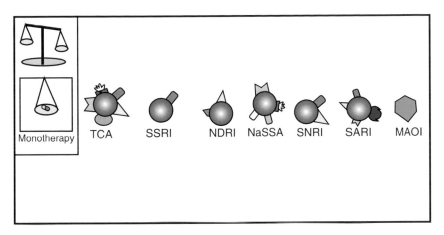

Monotherapy   TCA   SSRI   NDRI   NaSSA   SNRI   SARI   MAOI

FIGURE 7.2   The seven major antidepressant mechanisms of action are shown here. They include the classical tricyclic antidepressants and MAO inhibitors. Newer agents include SSRIs, dual serotonin and norepinephrine reuptake inhibitors (SNRI; e.g., venlafaxine), serotonin 2 antagonist/reuptake inhibitors (SARI; e.g., nefazodone), and in the USA, a norepinephrine and dopamine reuptake inhibitor (NDRI; bupropion). The seventh mechanism is NaSSA, namely Noradrenergic and Specific Serotonergic Antidepressant, exemplified by mirtazapine, and acting by dual enhancement of both serotonin and norepinephrine neurotransmission. This is mediated by alpha 2 antagonist properties. Tolerability is improved by additional 5HT2 and 5HT3 antagonist properties. See Figure 7.1 for additional explanation.

Table 7.1	MATCHING PATIENT PROFILES WITH ANTIDEPRESSANT DRUG PROFILES	
Patient profiles	*Antidepressant drug profiles*	*Examples*
atypical (weight gain; hyper-somnia; hyperphagia; anergia)	activating by 5HT or DA/NE	SSRIs, MAOIs, bupropion (USA)
anxious	5HT2 antagonist	nefazodone mirtazapine
agitated	5HT2 antagonist	nefazodone mirtazapine
insomnia	5HT2 antagonist	nefazodone mirtazapine
sexual dysfunction	5HT2 antagonist	nefazodone mirtazapine
	non-5HT	bupropion (USA)
pain	5HT2 antagonist/ 5HT reuptake	amitriptyline nefazodone? mirtazapine??
migraine prophylaxis	5HT2 antagonist/ 5HT reuptake	amitriptyline nefazodone? mirtazapine??
panic disorder	5HT	SSRI
obsessive compulsive disorder	5HT	SSRI
bulimia/binge eating disorder	5HT	SSRI

Rather than choose an antidepressant randomly, the prescriber can first profile the patient according to the features in the first column. By understanding pharmacologic mechanisms of action of the various antidepressants, a match can be made based upon the different drugs' profiles (middle column). Specific examples of the match are given in the third column. There are no hard and fast rules.

Table 7.2   ARE TWO MECHANISMS BETTER THAN ONE FOR SOME PATIENTS?

- rapid onset of antidepressant effects?
- severe depression?
- retarded depression?
- treatment resistant depression?
- melancholic depression?
- inpatient depression?
- dual action clomipramine better than the single action SSRIs paroxetine or citalopram?
- dual action venlafaxine or mirtazapine better than single action fluoxetine?
- more research needed

Several single agents nevertheless have two actions: namely they increase both noradrenergic *and* serotonergic neurotransmission. Theoretical considerations of the monoamine hypothesis of depression (Figs 2.1 and 2.2) as well as some data suggest that such agents may be preferable to single agents for the clinical situations listed in this table.

Table 7.3   SINGLE MECHANISM VERSUS DUAL ACTION ANTIDEPRESSANTS

Single action agents		*Dual action agents*
Mostly NE	*Mostly 5HT*	*Both NE & 5HI*
desipramine (TCA)	SSRIs	clomipramine (TCA)
bupropion (USA)	nefazodone	venlafaxine
mianserin (Europe)		mirtazapine, MAOIs

Specific examples of single action antidepressant agents are given in the first two columns of this table: the first column shows agents acting predominantly to increase noradrenergic neurotransmission; the second column shows agents acting predominantly to increase serotonergic neurotransmission. Dual action agents are shown in the third column. Since they increase both serotonergic *and* noradrenergic neurotransmission, they may be preferable for the clinical situations listed in Table 7.2.

CHAPTER 8

ANTIDEPRESSANT COMBINATIONS AND AUGMENTATION STRATEGIES FOR DIFFICULT CASES

It has been said that there are three types of psychopharmacologists: those who can count and those who can't. This chapter is written for psychopharmacologists who can't count. That is, when a patient has an unsatisfactory treatment response, a second agent may frequently be necessary to add to the first antidepressant. Thus, two or more drugs are combined. This is becoming the rule rather than the exception in the treatment of depression, especially in psychiatric practices where patients with unsatisfactory responses to previous antidepressants may be concentrated.

If patients are treatment resistant with little or no response to single agents, the psychopharmacologist hopes to find two agents where the first plus the second creates a therapeutic outcome greater than either drug alone. This approach looks for a combination of agents where the whole is greater than the sum of the parts, or in other words, where 1 + 1 = 10.

If patients are intolerant to single agents, this may prevent adequate treatment trials, or may lead to noncompliance and relapse. In this case, the psychopharmacologist hopes to find two agents where the second agent cancels or at least mitigates the side effects of the first, or in other words, where 1 + 1 = 0.

This chapter is a series of visual lessons on practical tips in combining antidepressants to achieve these goals. The approach here utilizes rational strategies for creating these combinations through the proper mixing of pharmacologic mechanisms of action.

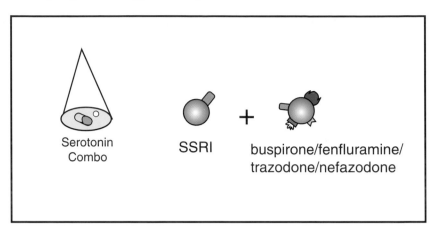

Serotonin Combo

SSRI

+

buspirone/fenfluramine/
trazodone/nefazodone

FIGURE 8.1. This figure depicts a 'serotonin combo', which represents a combination of serotonergic mechanisms listed in Table 8.1. The idea is to potentiate the action of serotonin reuptake inhibitors with a second serotonergic mechanism in order to boost the efficacy associated with the serotonin reuptake inhibitor alone. The serotonin strategy is depicted in Figures 8.1–8.14.

Table 8.1
The Serotonin Strategy

- Reuptake inhibition (SSRIs)
- 5-HT2 antagonism + SRI (nefazodone)
- 5-HT1A agonism (buspirone)
- 5-HT1A antagonism (pindolol)
- 5-HT release (fenfluramine)

One important strategy for combining antidepressants is to amplify serotonergic action using a combination of a serotonin selective reuptake inhibitor (SSRI) plus another serotonin augmenting agent. This can include a serotonin 1A receptor agonist (buspirone), a serotonin 1A antagonist (pindolol); a serotonin releaser (fenfluramine) or a serotonin antagonist/reuptake inhibitor (SARI)— (serotonin combos).

FIGURES 8.2–8.7.   Various serotonin combination strategies are depicted in Figures 8.2–8.14. If 5HT is depleted (Figure 8.2), adding an SSRI would have no effect (Figure 8.3) because there would be essentially no synaptic 5HT whose reuptake could be blocked.

Adding the 5HT1A agonist buspirone acts as a partial agonist at 5HT1A receptors (Figure 8.4), slowing neuronal impulse flow so 5HT can replete, and acting as a sort of 'artificial serotonin' causing 5HT1A autoreceptor down regulation. This may cause the neuron's serotonergic functioning to be sufficiently boosted that SSRIs can now act (Figure 8.5).

A similar action to that explained in Figures 8.4 and 8.5 has recently been proposed for pindolol. This agent is an antagonist of 5HT1A receptors in addition to its better known properties of beta receptor antagonism. If 5HT1A receptors are blocked by pindolol (Figure 8.6), this could cause immediate disinhibition of the serotonin neuron. Such actions may either cause faster-onset antidepressant action, or more satisfactory antidepressant action in refractory cases (Figure 8.7).

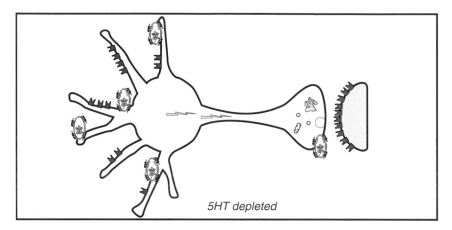

FIGURE 8.2

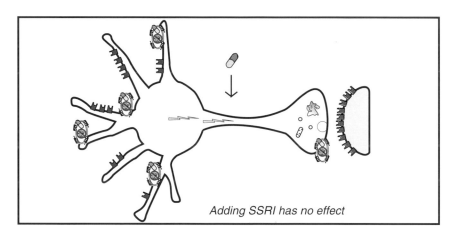

FIGURE 8.3

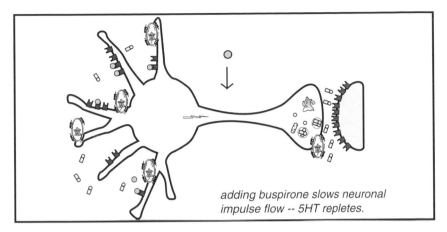

adding buspirone slows neuronal
impulse flow -- 5HT repletes.

FIGURE 8.4

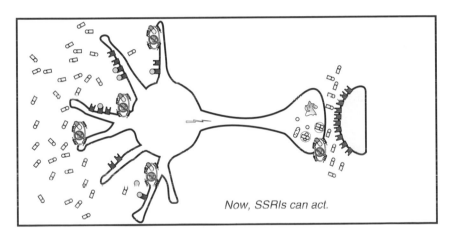

Now, SSRIs can act.

FIGURE 8.5

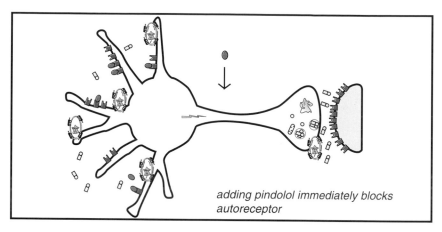

adding pindolol immediately blocks
autoreceptor

FIGURE 8.6

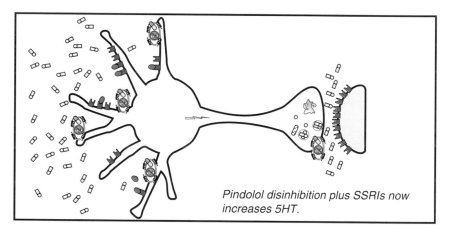

Pindolol disinhibition plus SSRIs now
increases 5HT.

FIGURE 8.7

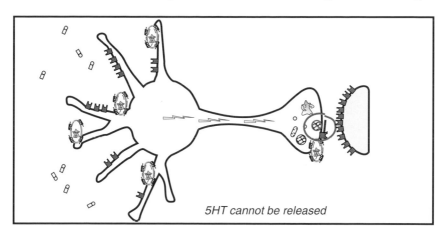

5HT cannot be released

FIGURES 8.8–8.10.   If 5HT cannot be released (Figure 8.8), a serotonin releaser such as fenfluramine (Figure 8.9) might be able to make 5HT available in the synapse. This approach much be taken with care, because too much serotonin release could theoretically be toxic (i.e., the 'serotonin syndrome' of fever, tremor, seizures, coma and even death). However, much more likely is the possibility that serotonin reuptake blockade will also block fenfluramine from having any action at all. Thus, fenfluramine and an SSRI may need to be given sequentially rather than concurrently. If successful, this approach might render SSRIs more effective (Figure 8.10).

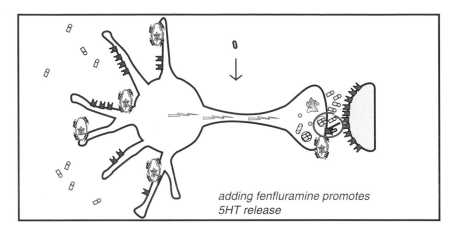

FIGURE 8.9

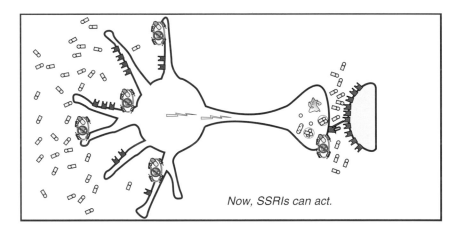

FIGURE 8.10

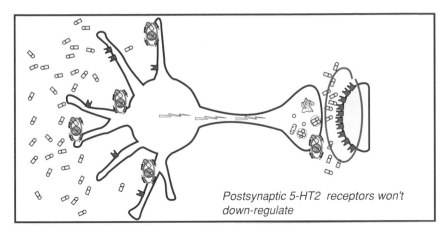

Postsynaptic 5-HT2 receptors won't down-regulate

FIGURE 8.11

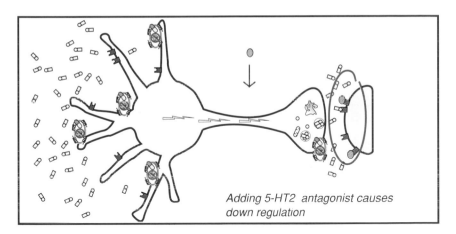

Adding 5-HT2 antagonist causes down regulation

FIGURE 8.12

FIGURE 8.11 and 8.12.   It is possible that SSRIs may not be able to effect a sufficiently robust down regulation of 5HT2 receptors (Figure 8.11). In that case, an independent mechanism of down regulation may be helpful, such as the co-administration of a 5HT2 antagonist to assist in the down regulation of 5HT2 receptors (Figure 8.12).

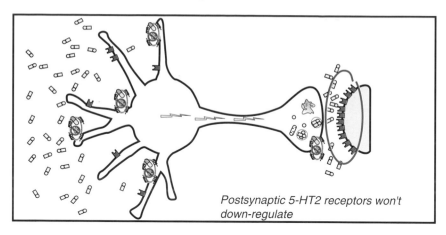

Postsynaptic 5-HT2 receptors won't down-regulate

FIGURE 8.13

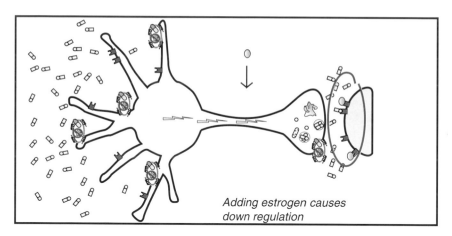

Adding estrogen causes down regulation

FIGURE 8.14

FIGURES 8.13 and 8.14.   In female rats, antidepressants cannot downregulate 5HT2 receptors if the ovaries are removed (Figure 8.13). However, if estrogen is administered, the ability of antidepressants to downregulate 5HT2 receptors is restored (Figure 8.14). This suggests that estrogen may be a useful adjunct for some perimenopausal and postmenopausal women who fail to respond adequately to antidepressants.

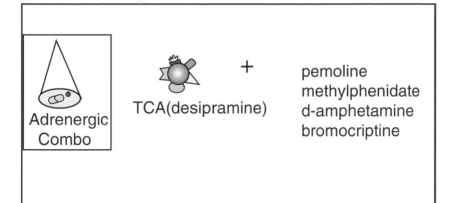

FIGURE 8.15. Another important strategy for combining antidepressants is to amplify adrenergic action by using a combination of a norepinephrine (noradrenaline) preferring tricyclic antidepressant with another agent which augments adrenergic function. Such noradrenergic augmenting agents can include dopamine agonists and dopamine releasers. Bupropion (USA) itself augments both norepinephrine and dopamine. Mianserin has predominantly noradrenergic actions – (adrenergic combos).

Table 8.2
The Noradrenergic Strategy

- Norepinephrine reuptake inhibition (desipramine, maprotiline)
- Dopamine and norepinephrine reuptake inhibition (bupropion)
- Dopamine agonists (bromocriptine)
- Dopamine releasers (pemoline, methylphenidate, amphetamine)

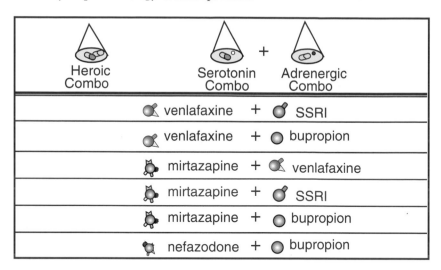

Heroic Combo	Serotonin Combo	Adrenergic Combo
	venlafaxine +	SSRI
	venlafaxine +	bupropion
	mirtazapine +	venlafaxine
	mirtazapine +	SSRI
	mirtazapine +	bupropion
	nefazodone +	bupropion

FIGURE 8.16. If augmenting a single neurotransmitter system is not adequate to produce an antidepressant effect, then augmenting both 5HT and NE neurotransmitter systems can be a powerful approach to the treatment of refractory depression (heroic combo).

As discussed in Chapters 5, 6 and 7, some agents such as clomipramine, venlafaxine and mirtazapine boost both 5HT and NE even as single drug agents. Thus, any of these can serve as a platform for superimposing other agents acting at 5HT, NE or both. Theoretically, one of the most powerful mechanisms to increase both NE and 5HT would be to combine mirtazapine with venlafaxine, thus boosting two neurotransmitters by two independent mechanisms, namely dual reuptake blockade plus dual disinhibition by alpha 2 blockade.

Table 8.3
The Serotonin Plus Adrenergic Combination Strategy

- Dual reuptake inhibitors (venlafaxine)
- TCA + SSRI (use caution)
- MAOI + TCA (use caution)
- Mirtazapine
- Clomipramine

CHAPTER 9

CYTOCHROME P450 AND ANTIDEPRESSANT DRUG INTERACTIONS

Recently there has been a veritable explosion in the understanding of the pharmacokinetic basis of drug interactions. Pharmacokinetics is the study of how the body acts upon drugs, especially to absorb, distribute, metabolize and then excrete them. Such pharmacokinetic actions are mediated predominantly through the hepatic drug metabolizing system known commonly as the cytochrome P450 hepatic enzyme system.

The cytochrome P450 enzymes and the pharmacokinetic actions they represent must be contrasted with the pharmacodynamic actions of drugs. In fact, this entire book has dealt almost exclusively with the pharmacodynamics of antidepressants, especially how antidepressants act upon the brain.

In the visual lessons which follow, the key enzymes which have important pharmacokinetic interactions with antidepressants drugs will be shown. Also, the consequences of these pharmacokinetic actions of antidepressants upon concomitantly administered drugs will be shown. This will lead to tips for avoiding unwanted drug interactions based upon an understanding of the pharmacokinetics of antidepressants and the cytochrome P450 enzyme system.

Table 9.1
PHARMACOKINETICS
How the body acts on drugs
PHARMACODYNAMICS
How drugs act upon the body (especially the brain)

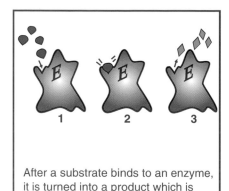

After a substrate binds to an enzyme, it is turned into a product which is then released from the enzyme.

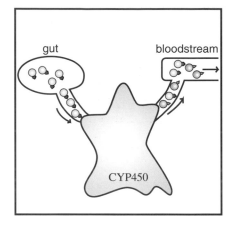

FIGURE 9.1. A substrate (1) interacts with an enzyme by binding to the enzyme's active site (2), and is transformed into a product (3).

FIGURE 9.2. Just as shown in Figure 9.1 for general principles of enzymes transforming substrates into products. Figure 9.2 shows how this occurs specifically in the cytochrome P450 enzyme system. That is, a drug ingested into the gut on the left serves as a substrate for a liver enzyme called P450. When the drug is absorbed and delivered to the liver, a biotransformation occurs so that the drug can eventually be excreted and eliminated from the body. Specifically, the biotransformation in the liver is for the P450 enzyme to convert the drug substrate into a biotransformed product in the bloodstream. After passing through the liver, the drug will exist partially as unchanged drug and partially as transformed product.

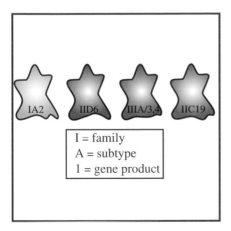

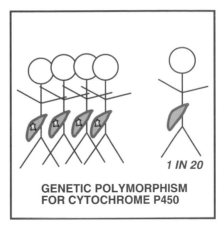

**GENETIC POLYMORPHISM
FOR CYTOCHROME P450**

FIGURE 9.3.   There are several known cytochrome P450 enzymes. Four of the most important for psychotropic drug metabolism are shown here. The first number is the cytochrome P450 family, then the subtype is indicated with a letter, followed by another number indicating the specific gene product which that cytochrome P450 enzyme represents.

There are over 30 known enzymes, and probably many more awaiting discovery and classification.

FIGURE 9.4.   Not all individuals have all the same cytochrome P450 enzymes. In such cases, the enzyme is said to be polymorphic. For example, about 1 in 20 caucasians lack the enzyme 2D6. They must metabolize drugs by alternate routes which may not be as efficient as the 2D6 route.

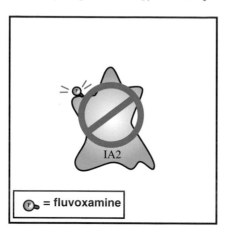

= fluvoxamine

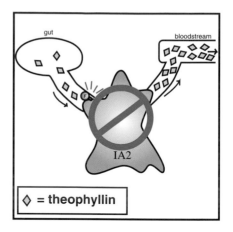

= theophyllin

FIGURES 9.5 and 9.6.   One Cytochrome P450 enzyme of relevance to psychotropic drugs is 1A2. This enzyme is inhibited by the SSRI fluvoxamine (Figure 9.5). Thus, when fluvoxamine is given concomitantly with other drugs which use 1A2 for their metabolism, those drugs can no longer be metabolized efficiently. An example of a potentially important interaction is when fluvoxamine is given along with theophyllin (Figure 9.6). In that case, the theophyllin dose must be lowered or else the blood levels will rise, and possibly cause side effects or even be toxic.

Table 9.2

The pharmacokinetic prevention of interactions

Part 1. Tips for avoiding 1A2 interactions

- Fluvoxamine may raise theophyllin and clozapine levels
- So could large amounts of grapefruit juice and the antibiotics ciprofloxacin and norfloxacin

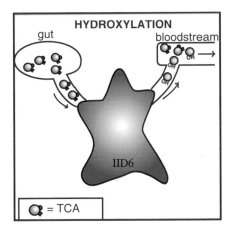

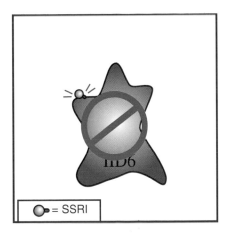

FIGURES 9.7, 9.8 and 9.9. Another cytochrome P450 enzyme of importance to prescribers of psychotropic drugs is the enzyme 2D6. This enzyme hydroxylates various drugs, including tricyclic antidepressants and mirtazapine (Figure 9.7).

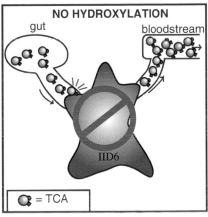

Several antidepressants are inhibitors of 2D6. This includes the SSRIs, although individual SSRIs differ in the potency of this effect from one to another (Figure 9.8). The importance of this is that when tricyclic antidepressants are given concomitantly with SSRIs, the plasma concentrations of the tricyclic antidepressant can rise, sometimes to toxic levels (Figure 9.9). Concomitant administration of an SSRI with a tricyclic antidepressant requires monitoring of the plasma drug concentrations of the tricyclic antidepressant, and possibly a dose reduction of the tricyclic antidepressant.

Table 9.3

The pharmacokinetic prevention of interactions
Part 2: Tips for avoiding 2D6 interactions
- SSRIs can increase TCA levels
- SSRIs can block the pain relief of codeine and raise codeine levels
- SSRIs can increase β-blocker levels

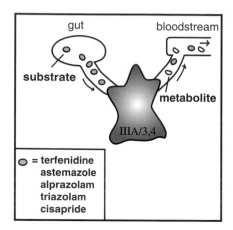

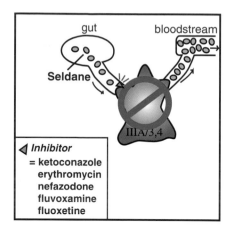

FIGURES 9.10 and 9.11. The cytochrome P450 enzyme 3A3,4 is a potentially important enzyme to all physicians. Several commonly-used drugs are metabolized by this enzyme (see Figure 9.10).

In some cases, the biotransformation of a 3A3,4 substrate drug is necessary in order to prevent a potentially toxic amount of the parent drug from accumulating in the plasma (Figure 9.11). This is exemplified by terfenadine, which is toxic if not biotransformed. If 3A3,4 is blocked by a powerful inhibitor, terfenadine can be fatal due to cardiac arrhythmia. The most significant inhibitors are the non-psychotropic agents ketoconazole and erythromycin. However several antidepressants are also weak inhibitors of this same enzyme (Figure 9.11).

Therefore, on theoretical grounds, nefazodone, fluvoxamine and perhaps even other SSRIs should not be co-administered with potentially toxic substrates of 3A3,4 (Figures 9.10 and 9.11) including not only terfenadine, but also astemazole, and cisapride. Other concomitantly administered substrates of 3A3,4 (such as alprazolam and triazolam) may need to have their dosages reduced when co-administered with the antidepressants which are inhibitors of 3A3,4 (such as nefazodone, fluvoxamine).

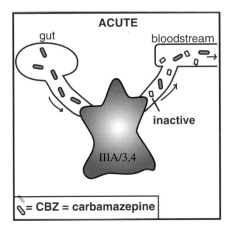

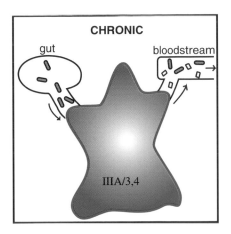

FIGURES 9.12 and 9.13.   Drugs can not only be substrates for a P450 enzyme, or an inhibitor of a P450 enzyme; they can also be inducers of a P450 enzyme and thereby increase the activity of that enzyme. One example of this is carbamazepine. This drug is both a substrate and an inducer of 3A3,4. Thus, when first starting carbamazepine, the levels of drug in the plasma will reflect the activity of the baseline, non-induced form of 3A3,4 (see Figure 9.12). Over time, however, the activity of 3A3,4 increases due to induction of this enzyme by carbamazepine. This can lead to reduction of carbamazepine levels, as the increased enzyme activity leads to more efficient metabolism of the substrate carbamazepine (Figure 9.13). To keep carbamazepine plasma levels constant, the dose may have to be increased to adjust for the autoinduction of 3A3,4.

Table 9.4

The pharmacokinetic prevention of interactions

Part 3: Tips for avoiding 3A3,4 interactions

- ketoconazole or erythromycin + terfenadine, astemizole or cisapride could be a dangerous or even lethal combination
- therefore, on theoretical grounds: avoid nefazodone, fluvoxamine and possibly fluoxetine and other SSRIs with these
- use loratidine, fexofenidine, cetinizine
- use lower doses of carbamazepine, alprazolam and triaolam as well
- carbamazepine can lower its own levels (autoinduction)

Table 9.5
Inhibition potential of the newer antidepressants at cytochrome P450 isozymes

Relative rank	Isozyme			
	1A2	2C19	2D6	3A4/4
High	Fluvoxamine	Fluoxetine Fluvoxamine	Paroxetine Fluoxetine	Nefazodone Fluvoxamine
Moderate	Fluoxetine	Sertraline	Sertraline	Fluoxetine Sertraline
Low-to-minimal	Paroxetine Venlafaxine Nefazodone Mirtazapine	Venlafaxine Mirtazapine	Venlafaxine Fluvoxamine Mirtazapine	Venlafaxine Paroxetine Mirtazapine

Table 9.6

Pharmacokinetics

Summary

- Many drug interactions are primarily of academic or marketing interest
- Many drug interactions are statistically significant yet clinically insignificant or easily managed
- Few combinations must be absolutely avoided
- Several combinations require dosage adjustment of one of the drugs.

INDEX

acetylcholine receptor 35
adrenergic combination strategy, plus
    serotonin 100
adrenergic 'combo' 99
alpha 1 antagonists 33, 36
    see also tricyclic antidepressants
        (TCAs)
alpha 2 antagonists 69
    see also mianserin
alpha 2 (hetero)receptors 20, 27
alprazolam, cytochrome P450 3A3,4
    substrates 106
amantadine 58
amitriptyline 65
amoxapine 38, 65
amphetamine
    noradrenergic strategy 99
    sexual dysfunction 58
anhedonia 56
anticholinergic antimuscarinic drug 33
antidepressants
    combinations and augmentation
        strategies 89–100
    complete armamentarium 84
    and cytochrome P450, interactions
        101–8
    downregulation hypothesis 8
    drug profiles, matching with patient
        profiles 86
    dual action vs single mechanism 87
    effects and time courses 6
    interactions
        avoiding Cy P450 3A3,4 interactions
            107

    summary 108
    seven major classes of action 85
    synergistic combinations 89–100
    upregulation hypothesis 7
antihistamine properties
    mirtazapine 77
    TCAs 35
anxiety, treatment 54, 86
appetite 57
aromatic amino acid decarboxylase,
        formation of serotonin 15
astemazole, with cytochrome P450
        3A3,4 substrates 106
autoreceptors 13, 17, 19

brainstem chemoreceptor trigger zone,
        nausea and vomiting 57
bromocriptine
    noradrenergic strategy 99
    for sexual dysfunction 58
bulimia, anti-bulimia action of SSRIs 51,
        86
bupropion
    clinical information 81
    mechanism of action 61, 80
    noradrenergic strategy 99
    preferred/least preferred uses 81
    for sexual dysfunction 58
    side effects 81
    structure 80
buspirone
    serotonin 1A receptor agonist 90, 93
    for sexual dysfunction 58

cancer chemotherapy, nausea and
vomiting, serotonin antagonists
action 57
carbamazepine, cytochrome P450
induction 107
catechol-O-methyl transferase
destruction of dopamine 14
destruction of norepinephrine 12
chemoreceptor trigger zone, nausea and
vomiting 57
ciprofloxacin 104
cisapride, with cytochrome P450 3A3,4
substrates 106
citalopram, classification 39
clomipramine, properties 38
clozapine 65
cyproheptadine 58, 65
cytochrome P450 101–8
1A2 reactions, avoiding 104
2D6 deficiency 103
2D6 hydroxylation of drugs 105
3A3,4
induction by drugs 107
metabolism of drugs 106
substrates 106
tips for avoiding interactions 107
and antidepressants, interactions
101–8
genetic polymorphism 103

deprenyl, classification 32
designer drugs 23, 71
desipramine
noradrenergic strategy 99
properties 38
dioxyphenylalanine *see* DOPA
DOPA, production 12
DOPA decarboxylase, action 12, 14
dopamine
agonists 99
destruction 14
dopamine-releasing drugs 99
neurotransmission 11

production 14
receptors, regulation of dopaminergic
neurotransmission 15
reversal of SSRI-induced sexual
dysfunction 56
dopamine beta hydroxylase, action 12
dopamine reuptake inhibitor (DRI) 80–1
see also bupropion
dopaminergic neurons, reuptake pump
14
downregulation
5HT2 antagonist 97
estrogen 98
hypothesis (antidepressants) 8
dual action drugs
vs single mechanism drugs 87
see also mirtazapine; tricyclic
antidepressants; venlafaxine

eating disorders 51, 86
estrogen, downregulation of 5HT2
receptors 98

fenfluramine, serotonin release 90, 95–6
fluoxetine
classification 39
clinical information 59
fluvoxamine
action 104
classification 39
clinical information 60
with cytochrome P450 3A3,4
substrates 106

gastrointestinal motility, SSRIs 24, 58
grapefruit juice 104

hepatic drug-metabolizing (cytochrome
P450) system, and antidepressants,
interactions 101–8
heroic 'combo' 100
5–hydroxytryptamine (5HT) *see*
serotonin

5-hydroxytryptophan, conversion to
    serotonin 15

insomnia
    SSRI-induced 55
    treatment 86
isocarboxazid, classification 32

ketoconazole, inhibition of cytochrome
    P450 3A3,4 106

lithium, mechanism of action 82

maprotiline
    noradrenergic strategy 99
    properties 38
methylphenidate
    noradrenergic strategy 99
    for sexual dysfunction 58
methysergide, migraine 65
mianserin
    disinhibition of noradrenergic neurons
        69
    mechanism of action 61, 69
    properties 69
migraine, methysergide 65
migraine prophylaxis 86
mirtazapine
    clinical information 79
        preferred/least preferred uses 79
        for sexual dysfunction 58, 86
    in combination
        with bupropion 100
        with SSRI 100
        with venlafaxine 100
    mechanism of action 61, 71
        direction of serotonin to 5HT1A
            receptor 76
        disinhibition of serotonergic
            neurons 69, 75
        post-synaptic NE-5HT interactions
            72
        pre-synaptic NE-5HT interactions 73

properties
    alpha 2 antagonist properties 73, 75
    antihistamine properties 77
    as designer (dual action) drug 71
    selective serotonin and
        norepinephrine (NaSSA) actions
        74, 78
    side effects 79
moclobemide, classification 32, 33
monoamine hypothesis of depression 4-5
monoamine oxidase, neurotransmitter
    destruction 4-5
monoamine oxidase inhibitors 31-3
    action 5, 8-9
    clinical information 33
    MAO A/B, reversible/selective
        inhibitors 32
    preferred/least preferred uses 32
    reversible (RIMAs) 31, 32
        action of NE 31
    side effect profile 32
monoamine receptor hypothesis of
    depression 6-7
myoclonus, slow wave sleep 55

NaSSA see noradrenergic and specific
    serotonergic antidepressant
nausea and vomiting, brainstem,
    chemoreceptor trigger zone 57
NE see norepinephrine
nefazodone
    with bupropion 100
    clinical information 68
    with cytochrome P450 3A3,4
        substrates 106
    mechanism of action 61, 66
    pharmacology 67
    preferred/least preferred uses 67-8
    for sexual dysfunction 58, 86
    side effects
        from 5HT2 blockade 67
        from MCPP metabolite formation 68
    structure 65

neurotransmitter{s} 11–28
neurotransmitter receptors
    downregulation 9
    theories of depression 6
    upregulation 7
noradrenergic and specific serotonergic
        antidepressant (NaSSA) 70–9
norepinephrine
    alpha 2 receptor 20
    blood pressure elevation 31
    disinhibition by mirtazapine 72
    interactions with serotonin 25–8
    normal production/destruction 12, 30
    reuptake inhibition (noradrenergic
        strategy) 99
    transporters 16
norepinephrine and dopamine reuptake
        inhibitor (NDRI) 80-1, 99
    see also bupropion
norfloxacin 104
nortriptyline 65

obsessive-compulsive disorder
    action of SSRIs 49
    treatment 86
olanzapine 65
    5HT2 receptor blockade 23

pain treatment 86
panic attacks
    raphe-limbic cortex pathway,
        serotonin disinhibition 50
    treatment 86
Parkinson's disease, dopamine receptors
    15
paroxetine
    classification 39
    clinical information 59
patient profiles, matching with drug
        profiles 86
pernoline, noradrenergic strategy 99
phenelzine, classification 32
phenylcyclopropaline, properties 33

pindolol, serotonin 1A receptor
        antagonist 90, 91, 94

refractory depression, heroic 'combo' 100
risperidone
    5HT2 receptor blockade 23
    serotonin 2 antagonist 65

SARIs see serotonin 5HT2 antagonist and
        reuptake inhibitors
schizophrenia, dopamine receptors 15
serotonin
    destruction by MAO 16
    neurons, disinhibition 18, 69, 75
    pathways in CNS 47
    plus adrenergic combination strategy
        100
    production 15
    release
        non-occupation of inhibitory
            receptors 21
        toxicity (serotonin syndrome) 95
    transporter, presynaptic transport
        pump 16
serotonin 'combo' strategy 90–8
serotonin 5HT2 antagonists
    in current psychiatric practice 65
    see also mianserin; nefazodone
serotonin 5HT2 antagonists and reuptake
        inhibitors (SARIs) 66–8, 90
    serotonin combination strategy 90–8
    see also nefazodone
serotonin receptors
    alpha 2 receptor, action 20
    autoreceptors 13, 17
    categories (subtyping) 16
    inhibitory receptors 20
    postsynaptic (5HT1A, 5HT1D, 5HT2A,
        5HT2C, 5HT3, 5HT4) 16
    postsynaptic (5HT1A)
        agonists 90
        pharmacology 18
        see also bupropion

postsynaptic (5HT2A)
  action 22
  antagonists in current psychiatric
    practice 65
  clinical tips 23
  clinically important consequences of
    blockade 65, 70
  production of second messengers
    22
  see also serotonin receptors
postsynaptic (5HT3)
  clinical tips 24
  clinically important consequences of
    blockade 70
presynaptic (5HT1A) 17
  clinical tips 18
  inhibitory action 20
  pharmacology 18
  stimulation, clinical consequences
    70
presynaptic (5HT1D) 16
  clinical tips 19
  inhibitory action 20
  pharmacology 19
serotonin selective reuptake inhibitors
    (SSRIs) 23, 39–60
  action
    consequences 44–6
    explanation 41–3, 48
    mechanism 43
    stimulation of 5HT2 and 5HT3
      receptors 52
  advantages/disadvantages 39–40
  clinical profile 48
  in combination
    with serotonin augmenting agent
      90–9
    with TCA, unblocking reuptake
      pump 34
  examples 39
  least preferred uses 60
  pharmacological profile 47
  serotonergic profile 74

side effects 24, 52
  akathisia and agitation 53
  anxiety and panic attacks 54
  gastrointestinal side effects 24
  insomnia 55
  sexual dysfunction 56, 58
therapeutic effects
  anti-bulimia profile 51
  anti-OCD profile 49
  anti-panic profile 50
  anxiolysis long-term 54
  clinical information 48, 58
  explanations 47
  tolerability 39
  see also serotonin antagonists and
    reuptake inhibitors
serotonin syndrome 95
serotonin-norepinephrine interactions
    25–8
  anatomical depiction 25–7
  excitatory 26
  inhibitory 27
  integrated model 28
  pre- and postsynaptic 25
serotonin-norepinephrine reuptake
    inhibitors (SNRIs) 62
  profiles 63–4
  see also venlafaxine
sertraline
  classification 39
  clinical information 59
sexual dysfunction
  recommended drugs 58, 86
  SSRI-induced 56, 58
single mechanism
  vs dual action drugs 87
  mostly 5HT *see* nefazodone; serotonin
    selective reuptake inhibitors
  mostly NE *see* bupropion; mianserin;
    tricyclic antidepressants
sleep
  brainstem centers, 5HT2 receptors 55
  slow wave, nocturnal myoclonus 55

smoking cessation 81
somatodendritic autoreceptors 17, 20, 44–6
SSRIs *see* serotonin selective reuptake inhibitors
synergistic combinations 89–100

terfenadine
  and cytochrome P450 3A3,4
    metabolism 106
  with cytochrome P450 3A3,4
    substrates 106
terminal autoreceptors 19
theophyllin 60, 104
theories of depression
  monoamine hypothesis 4–5
  monoamine receptor hypothesis 6–7
tranylcypromine, classification 32
trazodone
  insomnia 33
  mechanism of action 61, 66
triazolam, cytochrome P450 3A3,4
    substrates 106
tricyclic antidepressants (TCAs) 33–8
  action 5, 9, 34, 85
    explanation 37
    NRI portion in uptake pump 34
    SRI portion in uptake pump 34

clinical information 38
composition 33
norepinephrine-preferring 99
preferred/least preferred uses 37
side effects 35–6
  explanation 37
types 33
tryptophan, conversion to serotonin 15
tryptophan hydroxylase, action 15
tyramine
  action on norepinephrine 30
  effect of MAO 31
tyrosine, production of norepinephrine 12
tyrosine hydroxylase, action 12, 14

upregulation hypothesis
  (antidepressants) 7

venlafaxine
  clinical information 64
  least preferred uses 64
  mechanism of action 61–2
  pharmacology 63
  plus bupropion 100
  plus SSRI 100
  preferred uses 63
  side effects 63
  structure 62